W9-BUZ-808

Foundations of
HEALTH

ALSO BY DR. ERIC GOODMAN

Foundation: Redefine Your Core, Conquer Back Pain, and Move with Confidence

True to Form: How to Use Foundation Training for Sustained Pain Relief and Everyday Fitness

Foundations of
HEALTH

Harnessing the Restorative Power
of Movement, Heat, Breath, and the
Endocannabinoid System to Heal Pain and
Actively Adapt for a Healthy Life

DR. ERIC GOODMAN

FOREWORD BY JEFF BRIDGES

HARPER WAVE
An Imprint of HarperCollins*Publishers*

This book contains advice and information relating to health care. It should be used to supplement rather than replace the advice of your doctor or another trained health professional. If you know or suspect you have a health problem, it is recommended that you seek your physician's advice before embarking on any medical program or treatment. All efforts have been made to assure the accuracy of the information contained in this book as of the date of publication. This publisher and the author disclaim liability for any medical outcomes that may occur as a result of applying the methods suggested in this book.

FOUNDATIONS OF HEALTH. Copyright © 2022 by Eric Goodman. All rights reserved. Printed in the United States of America. No part of this book may be used or reproduced in any manner whatsoever without written permission except in the case of brief quotations embodied in critical articles and reviews. For information, address HarperCollins Publishers, 195 Broadway, New York, NY 10007.

HarperCollins books may be purchased for educational, business, or sales promotional use. For information, please email the Special Markets Department at SPsales@harpercollins.com.

FIRST EDITION

Designed by Nancy Singer

Library of Congress Cataloging-in-Publication Data has been applied for.

ISBN 978-0-06-299607-7

22 23 24 25 26 LSC 10 9 8 7 6 5 4 3 2 1

To my wife and only Sun.
To close family and friends.
To the students who have helped me share
Foundation Training.

With appreciation for what I got wrong, finding what felt right.

Contents

Foreword

Wow, Dr. Eric Goodman's new book, *Foundations of Health*, is a comprehensive and fascinating read that explores the connection between the mind and body.

I was fortunate to meet Eric, or "Air" as I call him, back in 2009, while I was working out with a fellow named Peter Park in Santa Barbara preparing for a movie. I was having terrible, debilitating back pain. I began working with Eric on my issues and his approach really helped me improve my overall health and strength. As a matter of fact, just recently, Eric told me he made his very first Foundation Training tape on my behalf, way back when.

Eric has spent years studying human physiology and movement and putting it into practice. He has helped me gain a better understanding of the physical, mental, and emotional aspects of being alive and how important it is to acknowledge these connections to heal. There are relatable metaphors throughout his book about pain in the body, which I found so interesting and inspiring. You may have a pain somewhere in your body that's not really being caused by the particular area where the pain is coming from. Learning to interpret the signals the body is giving, and how to respond to the signals, are important parts of well-being. The whole idea about pain being information, and reacting to that information properly, is the key to healing ourselves.

Let's say there's a light and it's not on so you think there's something wrong with the light. You can't figure out how to turn the light on. You're going to the bulb, you're looking at it until you realize that you've got to go over to the light switch on the wall. The light doesn't turn on where the light actually is, or where you think it should be, you have to go to its energy source to flip the switch. The body works in a very similar way.

I remember I had a gig, playing guitar with my band, The Abiders. My thumb was killing me. My whole hand and grip were just terrible. I couldn't bar a chord on my guitar. I called up Eric to see if he had any suggestions.

He said, "I'm going to tell you how to fix it right now. Find the sensitive spot in your elbow, put pressure on this point until it hurts, keep the pressure on it, and open and close your hand ten times."

I said, "No Eric, it's not in my elbow."

He said, "Listen to me, do what I'm telling you."

I did what he said to do, and *poof!* my pain was gone, no joke. All of a sudden, I could move my hand and play guitar.

The human body is amazing in its ability to heal itself, especially in stressful times. Eric expresses the importance of being curious about your physical conditions when presented, about how your body is reporting to you about the stress or situation. He helps us to dance with that stress. Life is a dance, man, and Eric is inviting you to join in. He encourages following the old saying "practice makes perfect." Just like playing a musical instrument and practicing, moving up and down the fret board, practicing and getting better. The human body is an instrument to train, practice, and manage until it becomes not second nature, but first nature in how you manage stress, recovery, and your health. It's all connected, man!

Eric continues to help me on many fronts with my physical health. He offers me mental and spiritual boosts with his knowledge. Eric's visionary approach to mindful movement and his teachings to harness the body's natural ability to heal is powerful. I am so grateful for Eric's guidance, friendship, and knowledge all of these years. He has helped me gain new insight, and he's given me the tools I use for a pain-free existence.

I encourage anyone who is interested in the connection between the mind, body, and healing to take a deep dive into Eric's work and to dance the dance of self-healing.

—Jeff Bridges

Introduction

I didn't arrive where I am today by design, I'll admit. I attended a traditional chiropractic school and was taught the standard subjects: anatomy and physiology, diagnosis and treatment. But as someone who actively seeks new information, who is deeply curious about the body, I never stopped learning. The more I learned, the more seemingly disparate protocols began to coalesce. The connections between different ways of healing just kept happening. Things I'd long suspected turned out to be true. Ideas I'd flirted with were suddenly justified in the latest scientific journals. Commonalities from patients' experiences began to make sense.

From all of this growing and connecting, all of these wanderings and discoveries, a unified theory emerged—one that focuses mostly on the concept of pain. I have come to realize that much of what we think we know about pain—what it means and how to treat it—is wrong. We fear and avoid the wrong things, and we look to the wrong places for solutions—which keeps us from finding immediate relief. Ultimately, it hampers us from living healthy lives in the long term. In the fifteen years I've been treating patients, my definition of what pain is—indeed, of what health looks and feels like—has evolved dramatically. It's grown more expansive, encompassing a wider and wider range of disciplines. Based on personal experience, sage advice from my peers, stories from my patients, and the latest scientific research, I've developed a theory of why things go wrong in our bodies and what we need to do to not only fix those things but to potentially prevent them from happening in the first place. I was thrilled when everything came into focus and I could pass on my wisdom to the people I treat; it's been transformative to my practice.

Foundations of Health is a great leap forward for me, moving beyond the standard terrain of biomechanics and spinal adjustments to incorporate other complementary modalities of care that, when employed together, can help you become pain free and set you on the path for a healthy, vibrant life. Some of these ideas have come to light relatively recently, so the exciting new science behind them is still emerging. But this journey started long ago, at a skateboard camp in Woodward, Pennsylvania, when I was only fifteen years old.

LEARNING FROM PAIN

In the summer of 1996, at Camp Woodward, an action sports camp in Pennsylvania, I dislocated my shoulder for the first time. Even after surgery, the injury meant I could no longer play hockey, which was my greatest passion and which I had planned to pursue in college.

As devastating as it was to have that future foreclosed, the loss also led me to an opportunity to shift, to grow in a radically new way. The one bright spot in my rough postsurgical recovery (twelve weeks in a brace) was rehabilitation with a gifted physical therapist named Chris. He taught me how my shoulder actually worked, explaining why my tendons had torn and how stabilizing the shoulder would relieve the pressure. He ended up fundamentally changing how I thought about the human body.

From there, Chris introduced me to weight training, and after I had worked with him for a year, *both* my shoulders felt more powerful than they had before I was injured. He showed me what it feels like when the support system around a joint or an injury is protected through strength. And he didn't just teach me what to do, he taught me *why* I needed to do it, the theory behind the practice. I felt better than I ever had, and I knew instinctually that I probably hadn't needed that operation as much as I needed the right kind of strength training to solve for that particular injury.

This was more than just the beginning of my journey with pain. My damaged shoulder and subsequent rehab led to the most intense spark of curiosity I had ever felt. I was connecting what I knew (my own sensations of pain and strength) with what I didn't know but very much wanted to (how the human body works). As I would come to realize, experience is the only way I know how to learn, and it's the only way I know how to teach: by leaning into what we feel in our own bodies and lives. Instead of running away from pain, I learned to listen to it and let it teach me something. That listening is at the heart of my entire philosophy.

To further follow up on these early lessons, I decided to become a doctor of chiropractic medicine, the field that teaches the most about the structure, form, and function of the human body. Three years into the program, though, I developed chronic back pain so severe that I almost quit.

The pain had been steadily creeping up on me. Playing ice

hockey and doing in-line skating led to early back stiffness. Then came years of swimming, diving, water polo, and lifting weights that further compressed my spine. I'd been trying to manage it by taking various painkillers and getting myofascial massages, physical therapy, and chiropractic adjustments. But it had become so bad that I knew if I went to the gym, I would hardly be able to walk the next morning. The seven A.M. drive to school hurt, as did sitting for eight hours a day in a classroom.

By my third year, I was actively seeing patients. The irony of treating people for the very same symptoms I was unable to address in myself was not lost on me. By the time I was twenty-seven, the pain and intensity were so severe that I turned to a group of doctors who specialized in back issues. An MRI showed major degeneration of most of my lumbar vertebrae, the worst being L4, L5, and the upper sacrum at the base of the spine. My bottom two vertebrae, the L5 and S1, were sitting directly on top of each other. No wonder I was in so much pain.

My doctors agreed that I needed two-level fusion surgery. They told me they'd stop the sacrum and last lumbar vertebrae from grinding against each other by grafting bone to my spine and fusing them together. The L4 would also be included in the circumferential bridge, to create additional relief and stability. It sounded like a drastic but effective solution. I dug into the medical literature and learned that there was a 20 percent chance the procedure wouldn't work. Plus, there was a risk that the operation would cause even more severe problems. I also couldn't help feeling that this course of action would be a betrayal of what I'd worked for. I'd spent years studying to become a chiropractor, which is a profession aimed at managing and healing musculoskeletal issues without surgery.

I was still young and athletic. Why was my body experiencing such frequent pain? Why was I being told my twenty-seven-year-old spinal discs were as worn as those of an old man? I was an aspiring doctor who had committed my life to understanding our musculoskeletal system. I must have missed something big to be feeling this bad.

I decided that I had to at least try to figure out what was going wrong, and to explore whether there was a legitimate nonsurgical solution. I knew that meant thinking beyond what I was learning in school. Truth be told, I was often frustrated during class. I never understood why anyone thought just realigning the spine without addressing the muscles that support it was a satisfactory long-term solution to anything. I learned that basic lesson from the physical therapist who helped me with my shoulder. Why wouldn't the same apply to my back health?

FINDING FOUNDATION

It took some time and a whole lot of trial and error, but eventually I recognized something fundamental. I was moving incorrectly. We all are.

More specifically, we move in ways contrary to how our bodies are constructed to move. Many of us endure chronic pain because of it. In our modern age, when so much of our time is spent sitting and staring at screens, our instincts have failed us. Since we aren't given an operating manual for our bodies, I set out to create one of my own.

I began rehabilitating myself, exploring varied flexion and extension exercises, sometimes further injuring my back along the way. Each of those brief self-inflicted pains helped me understand how localized sensation connected to the rest of my body. That insight eventually developed into a unique form of biomechanics—i.e., a series of postures, poses, and movements designed to teach individual muscles to act within strong, flexible chains of muscles. To my delight, it worked. My pain subsided, my mobility increased, and I learned to move my body in more natural ways. I made sure what I was doing was truly effective and long-lasting before I told my doctors that I appreciated their diagnosis but was passing on the surgery.

In healing myself, I learned that by training your posterior muscle chain—shoulders, back, butt, and legs—to share the burden of support, you take the obligation of force absorption away from joints and toward these large muscle groups. This allows you to disperse weight more evenly and maintain your alignment, even under stress. In addition to strengthening the muscles, these poses elongate and actively decompress your spine, create space between your well-stretched muscles, help to anchor your pelvis, and greatly ease your movement. All of these insights eventually turned into Foundation Training.

Based on these experiences and protocols, I wrote my first book, *Foundation* (2011), and another book after that, *True to Form* (2016). These books explain the biometric techniques that I developed and the movement and chiropractic principles behind them.

PART OF THE CURRENT

I was evangelical about my new ideas. Indeed, how could I not be? I had fixed myself and was having terrific success using these new techniques in healing my patients. One of the greatest pleasures it brought me was a community of like-minded people—professionals who worked in pain management or physical therapy or chiropractic medicine at the forefront of their fields. Those people introduced me to the work of other thinkers and writers, and my understanding and base of knowledge kept expanding. I started listening more and talking less. I realized I was substantially more valuable as part of this group than I was on my own. I was no longer interested in trying to prove the theory behind Foundation Training. I knew it worked, but now I wanted to understand how it could work in conversation with other people's ideas about health and pain management.

I began thinking of my work as part of a strong current sweeping us toward wellness.

There are so many ways to get better, to be healthy. We are all working toward the same goal, and there is no one right way to achieve it. The only thing you must do is plunge into the current. Look around and be open to learning and experiencing new things.

For over a decade now, I have been soaking in what experts in related areas of health have been doing, paying careful attention to what has and hasn't worked for me and for my patients, and exploring the evolving science underneath it all. I've opened myself up to a whole host of new practices and modalities to complement and enrich my training. And I have also come to see, in my patients' lives and my own, that the ongoing project of working toward emotional and mental wellness is just as important as any physical regime. There is an essential synergy between these two kinds of work, and that's become a cornerstone of my approach.

LEARNING FROM PATIENTS

This evolution of my thinking could not have been possible without my patients. For the past ten years, I have surrounded myself with people who have pushed the boundaries of the work we are doing together. They have done far more than improve their own physical and mental selves. Their struggles and insights have contributed to a unique collective wisdom that resonates widely and that others can learn from. Just as a body works within a system—and it's important to heed the whole system—our body of knowledge benefits from shared systems as well. What I first intuited, then honed on myself, and eventually shared with patients comes full circle when shared as a community to complete our understanding about how these practices can work to heal us.

In this book, you'll meet some of these patients and hear their stories. Seychelle Webster is a champion paddleboarder whose debilitating neck injury forced her to retrain her body and rethink her definition of strength. Josh Holland is a top-notch trainer and biohacker who has learned to treat his own severe scoliosis, believe it or not, with breathing. Surfer and waterman Erik Antonson and I developed protocols for him to manage the debilitating pain of spondylolisthesis without surgery. Tony Blauer, a master in the self-defense community, faced challenges that stretched the level of injury that Foundation Training could address. Jackson Fortunato came to Foundation Training terrified that his injuries might sideline his jiujitsu career. After a lifetime of hard-core sports, Patti Sheaff, a legend in the California surfing community, was broken down in more ways than she could count, but dedicated to remaining well enough to do the things she loves. Firefighter Evan Halquist has been applying the principles of Foundation Training to strength training and turning an ever-growing number of his fellow firefighters on to our work.

You'll also hear directly from folks who aren't patients but who have a wealth of expertise and knowledge that has enriched my work and my thinking in this book. Pat Helma is a chiropractor who's become a vital sounding board and a wise part of the Foundation team. Alli Cost's experience as a pediatric occupational therapist has revolutionized how I think about the ways in which Foundation Training can be applied to younger patients. Ben Carraway's understanding of the neurology of stress and the process of adaptation has become a backbone for Foundation Training theory.

Throughout the book, I'll turn to Jessie Salas, whom I've known since I was twenty-one. Jessie's immediate and complete immersion in Foundation Training has imbued it with fresh energy, strength, and commitment since 2014. He is a gifted, inspiring coach who has brought our work into new arenas. Jessie retired from a decorated seventeen-year firefighter career in order to lead Foundation Training into Fire Fighting and First Responder health initiatives, as well as develop the Baseline Strength program. Jessie and I share the role of co-leader in our Instructor Education Courses.

Foundations of Health presents, for the first time, my theory for holistic self-healing and incorporates treatments that work powerfully in conjunction with Foundation Training biomechanics. It is the culmination of fifteen years of daily research and experience but also of listening intently to the people I've treated and using their experience to expand the way I approach my work. I'm excited to share this next evolution of Foundation Training and hope that you find it a powerful guide for enhancing your life.

Foundations of
HEALTH

CHAPTER 1

Pain and Healing: A New Understanding

WHAT IS PAIN?

The body is a vastly complex ecosystem, an environment of linked systems that interact symbiotically and synergistically. Each of our body's main processes, from digestion to circulation and respiration, work in concert to keep the whole body functioning, balanced, and healthy. Our blood carries digested nutrients and oxygen from the lungs to cells across the body, including in our bones, which in turn create new blood cells. Our musculoskeletal system creates a protective cage around organs like the liver and kidneys, which rid the body of waste produced by (among others) bone cells. Muscular contractions in the digestive tract and movement in the skeletal system create healthy digestive, lymphatic, and immune systems. Healthy breathing improves muscular flexibility, circulation, and lymphatic drainage, which improves our immunity. All of our parts work together to create a thriving whole.

Seeing those intersystemic connections involves holding a lot of complex ideas together at once, and that is no small task. Nowhere is this challenge clearer than in the way we understand pain. Our conventional medical approach most often looks at pain as something local, something that exists only at the place that hurts the most. For example, if your wrist hurts, your wrist is the problem. If you have a headache, then you must have a problem in your head. Back pain means you have something wrong with your spine. So we treat the immediate location of the pain instead of its source. This really doesn't work.

Our understanding of pain is best comprehended—and treated—when we consider it in the context of the whole body. Seen this way, the real answers are more complex: that wrist pain might be the result of stimulated nerves in the spine or neck. That headache might be the result of untreated scalene (neck) inflammation, perhaps even digestive dysfunction or a chronically clenched jaw. That back problem might be the result of a hip or knee injury causing you to overcompensate and put too much pressure on the lower back. From this point on, I want you to understand that pain constitutes information and we are going to learn how to harness that information toward healing.

The big picture here is that chronic pain is often not a localized issue at all. It is a failure in the ecosystem, a breakdown somewhere in the relationships between the body's various systems. The symbiosis and synergy that should be happening is interrupted, and that failure ripples out well beyond its point of origin. Pain may result from a purely mechanical or neurological breakdown, but it could just as easily be a block in the communication between two systems.

Consider headaches again, for instance. Of course, some are caused by a musculoskeletal response, from sleeping wrong or whiplash. But many headaches are a digestive and lymphatic issue: there's something in our guts that shouldn't be there, and the body is responding with inflammation during its attempts to purge.

I have come to define pain as some kind of interruption of flow, and that flow can involve any tissue in the body. Pain can manifest itself in so many ways that if you're just reacting to the symptom—the sore knee, the frozen shoulder—you aren't listening to what your body is trying to tell you. This is of course frustrating, because we all want a definitive diagnosis, and in some ways, it's much easier to think about just fixing your elbow or addressing the pain in your neck. While some exercises will help alleviate these issues, I have found that the better, more long-lasting fix seems to lie in improving the intersystem relationships within the body. When these systems learn to communicate more effectively and efficiently, the body no longer needs to send out a distress signal, and pain vanishes.

Here's another example from my own life. Since middle school I've had digestive issues that would come and go, a low-grade irritable bowel syndrome that flared up occasionally, causing discomfort. This never got so bad that it had a huge impact on my physical health, but it absolutely affected my state of mind. Despite constantly chasing the perfect diet, I couldn't digest food easily, and I was often tired. This became more of an issue for me in graduate school, when I was under stress and sitting in class eight hours a day. If you remember, it's also when the pain in my back had reached a crisis point. I knew from the X-rays that my lower back—my L4,

L5, and S1—was my worst injury. That's right where your spine meets the sacrum, which then connects to the pelvis.

You know what's right in front of that? The sigmoid region of the large intestine, the same digestive tissue that had been mildly irritating me for over a decade. One of the biggest changes that I noticed with Foundation Training over the years was a radical improvement in my digestion. At the time, I was focused on my spine injury, trying to create space around and strength in the damaged bones and tissue. But it turns out that creating that space had an enormous impact on my digestive health. The improvement in my digestion was directly correlated with more energy and creativity and a greater sense of well-being. Every single one of those things improved as my back, and then my digestion and elimination, became healthier.

If I had gone to a doctor for my low-grade bowel issue, they would have examined my diet, looked for any blockages or physical issues, and most likely ended up prescribing an antacid or NSAID to help with inflammation. Few practitioners would have correlated digestive health with back pain, and even I didn't make the connection at the time. But now that's how I view every symptom I am presented with in my own body, as well in those of my patients. Every focal point of pain tells a larger story, and as our first patient found out, if we aren't listening to that larger story, we have no chance of adequately addressing the pain.

AVOIDING THE TRADITIONAL PATH

Sixty-four-year-old Patti Sheaff is a passionate lifelong surfer who for the past ten years has been evolving away from a "call the doctor/

treat the injury" approach to her pain. But it's important to remember where she started.

Patti Sheaff, Surfer

I took a fall snowboarding in 2010 and shattered my sacrum. That was the turning point, the start of probably four years—maybe more—of a lot of agony, a lot of trying to figure out how to get strong. Just dealing with the pain was my main objective at that point. I was athletic—still surfing—but just in so much pain I couldn't pick my surfboard up off the ground.

I worked for UCLA for a good part of my life, so I had decent health insurance. I had epidurals, a little microsurgery, and then I found RFAs, which are radiofrequency ablation, a procedure where they go in and burn all the nerves on your spine. I had maybe nine epidurals throughout those four years, and two or three RFAs, and the microsurgery. Some of them helped with the pain, but I was also on Percocet for about three or four years. It meant I could surf and play, but then six months later, the pain would come back—that's how it works.

On top of that, I've got pretty major scoliosis, and lots of back pain because of it. To tell you the truth, it was never really addressed. An orthopedic guy tried to give me orthotics, but you know, I don't wear shoes, so that didn't work. I even tried to glue flip-flops together, and it was just ridiculous. Chiropractic care worked for me for a long time. Until it didn't. It was an overnight thing, he just stopped being able to get any movement out of my lower spine.

Patti's lifestyle may be out of the ordinary, but her experience of pain is in fact quite normal. You may have never stepped on a surfboard or gone snowboarding (let alone skydiving, Patti's other passion), but the truth is, you have most likely been in pain or will be at some point. Eighty percent of people in the United States alone will experience back pain at some point in their lives. That's not to speak of the many other pain points and issues. I say this not to scare you, only to point out that chronic pain is a true epidemic in this country, and the way it's traditionally been addressed is only making things worse.

I have heard a variation of Patti's story from almost every patient I've seen over the past several years. There is an injury or constant discomfort, followed by X-rays and MRIs, an official diagnosis that sounds terrifying, physical therapy, and often surgery. Almost without exception, this is the path we set down when we wake up with back pain, or when hours spent on the computer have resulted in carpal tunnel syndrome or looking down at our phones constantly has caused neck strain.

The first warning sign you get that your body is out of alignment is usually back pain. Whether it's fallout from a strenuous session at the gym or just weeks of vague tightness and discomfort, your body is trying to tell you that something is wrong. You go to your doctors, and they run some tests. More often than not, they are going to find something—a bulging disc, a herniation, disc degeneration, arthritis. Now they have something to focus on, something to treat. As we saw with Patti, physical therapy, pain pills, and operations soon follow.

The major mistake here is that from the outset, the focus becomes too narrow. Along with a disconnected/segmented approach to pain comes a "quick fix" mentality for solving it. Just like we might head to the drive-through when we're hungry, we take Advil for a headache, get an epidural for back pain, or endure surgery for a herniated disk. If we just surgically repair that knee or shoulder or hip, we think, we'll be as good as new in a few months. The quicker we can get out of pain, the better.

The problem is that quick localized fixes often don't work, particularly over a long period of time. Steroid injections might ease chronic lower back pain temporarily, but as Patti will sadly remind you, the effects wear off after just a few months, and then you're back to where you started, ready to try something else. Spinal surgeries, the number of which increased 70 percent from 2001 to 2011 and continue to rise exponentially, are hugely popular, but clinical studies show most actually do not result in meaningfully better outcomes for patients than nonsurgical treatment. In fact, surgery might make things worse. One study used data from the Ohio Bureau of Workers' Compensation to look at the efficacy of spinal fusion surgery. Two years after the procedure, only 26 percent of patients returned to work and 41 percent were using more painkillers. Meanwhile, 67 percent of patients who did not have surgery had returned to work.

Painkillers themselves are an enormous part of the problem. Though opioids have become a standard prescription for back pain, we are now learning that they are actually ineffective and can even cause more pain, an effect called opioid-induced hyperalgesia. Rather than reducing pain messages to the brain, opioids (usually when taken in higher doses for a longer time) can do the opposite, causing increased pain sensitivity in the nervous system, to both existing and new injuries or conditions. On top of that, the frequency and recklessness with which opioids have been given to patients has caused a major epidemic in this country, claiming nearly 69,710 lives in 2020 alone, up nearly 18,000 from the previous year.

Instead of thinking of the symptom in isolation, as something just to be treated, we have to start thinking about symptoms as a road map. The herniation, the bulging disc, the pain, and repetitive stress injuries that we endure are all pointing to a larger issue: they are often products of poor movement patterns over time.

One of our Foundation Training practitioners, Alli Cost, who is also an occupational therapist, is often helping her patients create that road map, moving them away from siloed thinking. When an avid gardener came into her office complaining of severe carpal tunnel syndrome, the first thing Alli asked was to see what position she gardened in. The patient balked: "You're not doing anything for my wrist." So Alli drew a picture to show her how a pinched nerve in the back might be felt in the wrist. "People tend to look at the tree," she says. "So when I explain that we're looking at the entire forest, sometimes I need to draw them a little path so they can see how to get through it themselves."

When you tear the anterior cruciate ligament (ACL) or the posterior cruciate ligament (PCL) in your knee, your first impulse is to treat the ligament in isolation—with surgery. But when you step back and look at what's around that ligament, you realize that developing the muscles of the hamstrings, the sartorius (which runs down the length of the thigh), and the adductors (muscles that run along on the body's inner edges, extending and wrapping from the hip to the back of the femur, just in from where the glutes attach) in the right way can be a far more effective long-term solution to knee stability. Consider the muscles that connect at a point just below the inside knee called the pes anserinus. The tendons of three important support muscles for the knee—the sartorius, the gracilis, and the medial hamstring—all converge here. Without the support of these muscles, the knee is relying only on itself. All this is to say that the stability and health of a joint is a muscular obligation.

Our bodies are very good at sending us warning signs that something isn't right. These warning signs come in the form of the common complaints that we have—back pain, headaches, hip pain, plantar fasciitis, shin splints. Once we get a warning sign like that, we face a choice. Do we head to the doctor for a quick, temporary fix? Or do we pay attention to the pain more closely, put it in the context of an ecosystem, work harder to feel out the connections for ourselves?

THE BIGGER PICTURE

Understanding pain fully requires more than looking at connections between the systems of the body in a narrowly anatomical way. It's also about looking at how the body interacts with the mind. While structural issues need to be addressed (we'll get into that in the next chapter), it's equally important to examine the mental component to chronic pain as well.

Back in the throes of my increasing back issues, in early 2006, I decided to finish up chiropractic school in California, which unfortunately meant a cross-country drive. I was listening to back-to-back Howard Stern episodes to pass the time when I first heard Dr. John Sarno. Howard himself had been racked with debilitating back pain for years. It got so bad he had to lie down during commercial breaks to try to ease the pressure on his spine. He was, no surprise, scheduled for surgery when someone told him to see Dr. Sarno. Who was this guy that Howard called his personal hero, "the Steve Jobs of pain management" and the person who "saved his life"? It turns out that Sarno's idea was pretty simple. Pain is mostly in your head.

Sarno developed what he called tension myositis syndrome (TMS) to explain the psychosomatic condition that produces pain—mostly lower back pain, but also neck and shoulder pain, headaches, and even stomach and digestive issues. He determined that in the absence of something objectively, physically wrong, the pain that people felt was a result of repressed psychological or emotional issues. The brain, in an effort not to face the anger or tension or fear you are really feeling, manufactures pain as a way of distracting you from these negative emotions.

This does not mean the pain isn't real. It's very real. It just isn't necessarily caused by a bulging disc or early onset arthritis or whatever diagnosis your doctor may have given you. Instead, it can be caused by the fact that your body responds to the stress of pain by tensing up or breathing shallowly, all of which can create a cascade of secondary pain. Or, as Sarno suggests, pain may simply be created by your nervous system to give you something to focus on.

That's a pretty radical statement for a medical doctor with degrees from the most prestigious schools. Since the idea flew in the face of conventional medicine, Sarno was mostly ignored or outright mocked by his peers. Yet he helped countless people alleviate their suffering. No wonder Stern called him a hero. Sarno believed that once patients knew this pain was just a symptom—not of a structural issue, but of an emotional issue—they had the power to overcome it. Not only is that a major shift in how to think about pain, but it also empowers patients with their own cure. What a far cry from taking drugs or relenting to surgery.

Sarno's advice was to tackle the emotional issues that were throwing your life off-balance. He suggests that instead of lying in bed or taking pills or passively visiting a chiropractor, you should be active-walking and exercising as much as you comfortably can. Sarno was completely ahead of his time when he first began treating patients based on his theory.

At this point, you are probably thinking, as I was, what about those very terrifying-looking X-rays that showed spinal compression or herniated discs? Isn't that some sort of objective truth? The answer is yes. You may have some physical abnormalities. But that doesn't mean they are actually causing pain. Sarno would argue that there are plenty of people with exactly the same X-ray results who are *not* in pain, as well as plenty of people in pain whose X-rays reveal no structural issues whatsoever. Pain felt is real pain, no matter its cause, and we have to be open to understanding its primary source in order to overcome it. We have to learn to see it as part of a larger picture.

A 2007 peer-reviewed study showed a 54 percent reduction in the average pain intensity scores from fifty-one patients who had, before Sarno treated them, been in chronic back pain for an average of nine years. But the real proof comes in the testimonials of his patients—in Facebook groups, news programs, and even a documentary film devoted to his work, and person after person crediting Sarno's methods with saving their lives.

Sarno passed away in 2017 (at age ninety-three), but he would be very pleased to see that the medical establishment that shunned his work is coming around to agree with him. The idea of bed rest has gone by the wayside, and Sarno's concept of encouraging movement has become mainstream. But perhaps most important, while the majority of doctors are still trapped in the old way of thinking, there is increasing credence paid to the part our minds play in creating pain in our bodies. The mind-body connection—originally proposed by wisdom leaders of the past and philosophers/physicians of ancient cultures, and more recently thought to be the purview of practitioners of new age healing—has finally come full circle as a scientifically proven and necessary consideration for healing both our physical and mental selves. Sarno was there all along.

WHAT IS HEALING?

A broader definition of pain—as not just stemming from a localized injury, but as the result of a complex set of relationships within the body and between the body and the mind—offers us the opportunity to take control back from an antiquated health-care industry. It gives us the chance to define healing more broadly as something we can and must do for ourselves. As I have learned from my own and all of my patients' experiences, the true path to wellness demands autonomy.

At the heart of my broader do-it-yourself understanding of healing and wellness are a trio of interrelated concepts: curiosity, active adaptation, and resilience. I think of these not as static qualities or traits, but rather active processes to practice. Together they form the rationale that undergird and connect the specific treatment protocols that this book explores. Let's look at that rationale more closely.

CURIOSITY

As we've discussed, most of us have grown up with a passive attitude about our pain—indeed, about our own bodies more generally. The familiar sting or ache recurs, and we sigh with resignation, wondering how long it will last this time. We modulate our activities to lessen the occurrence and hope for the best, debating when to call a doctor, when to put our healing in the hands of someone else. But there is another way.

In order to begin to truly heal, we must come to understand that pain is a signal that needs to be interpreted. And we must shift our understanding about how to deal with pain from the conventional expectation that a cure will come from someone else or outside of ourselves, to realizing that we are in control of our own relief.

A key component of this journey is simple curiosity, specifically active engagement with sensation: pushing beyond fear and paralysis to inquisitiveness, moving from the statement "I don't know what's wrong with me" to the statement "What's going on here and how can I make it better?" There is a certain boldness to curiosity that I want to emphasize. It's not just asking questions, but also feeling out answers, acting on hunches, probing our own bodies in a deeper, fuller way.

The main process we are learning is somatosensation—the conscious perception of touch, pressure, pain, temperature, position, and movement that arises from the muscles, joints, and skin. Put a different way, it is how we assess what is happening to our bodies and within them. Somatosensation is a skill, a language, that we can develop. Related to somatosensation is proprioception—the understanding in our brains and bodies of how we take up and move through space. Do you stand with one hip higher than another? Are you constantly clenching your jaw? Do you sit with your shoulders slumped forward? We all have the ability to analyze what we are feeling and how we move through the world. But learning to do so requires strengthening the mind-body connection and actively employing a sense of curiosity about what we are feeling and why.

Pause for one moment here and ask yourself: How are you reading this book? Are you sitting up straight or hunched over? What is the position of your head? Are you lying down? Is your neck supported? Awareness of how we hold ourselves is important to understanding that we have more control than we think we do over how our bodies feel.

The relationship we have between mind and body is intimately tied to our sense of self-confidence and self-worth, and that relationship can deteriorate in different ways. If we carry around a lot of insecurity and doubt, that can translate into our feeling sluggish or weak. It can affect how we hold our bodies and postures. Trying to improve ourselves in this state feels overwhelming. We give up more often and can disconnect our mind from our body even further, until sensation becomes all-encompassing and indefinable. We have lost all somatosensation. "What's wrong?" someone might ask. "I hurt." Where? "All over." Why? "I don't know." What are you doing about it? "I take a pill. I see the acupuncturist." We literally lose the mind-body language, and we lose the curiosity necessary to look deeper.

Most of my first-time patients lack the skills to translate the sensations of the internal ecosystem of the body. Not only do they not know *why* they hurt, but they often have a hard time articulating where the hurt is coming from. I start by asking questions that they learn to ask themselves. This gives them the language necessary to pay closer attention and to help themselves. Ultimately this new language and awareness helps them to keep their bodies in positions that are efficient and feel good.

As you learn and practice somatosensation and proprioception, you will grow more curious, more willing to feel what is happening with your body and to actively break old patterns. With a healthier connection between mind and body, you'll see physical strain as something not to flinch from but to pursue in order to grow stronger.

In my own experience, curiosity is what led me to embrace the mental/emotional side of my own healing. At the time as I was treating my back through posture and movement, I was also becoming less fearful and more confident, intellectually and professionally. I was making my life less emotionally stressful, which helped me lessen physical stress as well.

Think of this as a process of self-study, of your learning what your body and your emotional state are trying to tell you. Other teachers and I will guide you in this process, but my hope is that with our help, you will be able to take charge of your own healing and need less help from us.

Once you've learned this new language of your body, you can and should practice it for the rest of your life. Along the way, you'll discover that the language of feeling itself changes and deepens, that there are always more nuances and layers to discover. On a broader level, the more you learn and explore, the richer your experience on this earth becomes.

So how exactly do we develop our somatosensation?

ACTIVE ADAPTATION AND STRESS

Bold curiosity is what compels us to, and then infuses, the next step: adapting actively; taking our capacity to change into our own hands. Every time someone else gets you better, you become a little more passive and dependent. Whereas in my work, any time you get *yourself* a little bit better, you become a lot more independent, starting on a path of healthfulness.

For us to embrace that process, though, we may need to unlearn a lot of what we've been taught and we might have to disregard a lot of things we've been told we cannot do. One thing I hear constantly from patients: "My doctor tells me I have the spine of an eighty-year-old!" I don't know who these doctors are or how many eighty-year-old spines they've seen, but that is not a helpful thing to tell anyone. If you think that your outcome is going to be dire or that you are powerless or that your pain is permanent, you are going to negatively affect your prognosis. Your healing process will succeed only if you think of what you *can* do with the body you have.

A lot of people blame the epidemic of chronic pain on some vague notion of the necessary stresses of modern life. "Commutes are killing our backs." "Computers are damaging our wrists." "Looking at screens is hurting our necks." "Sitting is the new smoking." Since this is what life will continue to entail for many of us, it might help to reframe what stress is. Just as we've learned that pain is not a localized event, something to be treated with a pill or an operation, stress is not something to be overcome or avoided. Whether we like it or not, we're all using phones and desks and cars, frequently putting our body into various compromised positions. The way I see it, modern life continually provides enough stress to ensure that we must respond to it well, physically and mentally. The stress is never going to change, so all we can change is how we are meeting the daily challenges that we encounter. And that means taking an active role in our adaptation.

We're adaptive creatures. That's the nature of all living beings. No matter what we do, we are stimulus-response organisms: until we die, we are adapting every day. Every single experience we have changes us, our mind or our body, whether we are aware of it or not. What we do with this extraordinary capacity to adapt is up to us. Every experience changes us, yes, but it can change us for good or for ill. We can embrace our adaptiveness with open arms, making sure we are adapting in ways that are healthy, both mentally and physically—that's active adaptation. Or we can just go along for the ride, giving into bad habits like poor posture, unhealthy food choices, or destructive thought patterns, making no effort to adapt positively—that's complacent adaptation.

Think of life as a dance and adaptation as your partner. You can let adaptation swing you around and wind up sprawled out in what-ever position you happen to end up in. Or you can learn to dance and participate in the process. Then when the dance changes, you can learn the steps of the new dance and keep on going. When the dance gets complicated and more demanding, you're ready to learn those moves, too—because active adaptation is a self-reinforcing process.

Here's an easy example of active adaptation. During the ubiquitous Zoom calls and teleconferences that dominate our lives, I've noticed that I have a tendency to cock my head to the right. Perhaps it's a sign of active listening, but it's also a bad habit that can result in strained neck muscles. Once I saw this was happening and felt it, I made a conscious effort to lengthen my neck, making sure the weight of my head was pushed back a little and properly balanced. Now, even without the visual cue, I can feel when my head is cocked, and I adjust it. After I've corrected my posture, say, twenty times, it becomes automatic, my body's preferred position. Because it feels better. Active adaptation is understanding your body is going to adapt, no matter what, and taking control so that it adapts in positive, healthful ways.

The age-old idea of creating positive, achievable mantras and healthy habits locates the power back with patients, ensuring they are taking an active, positive part in their own treatment. So when I work with patients with chronic pain, one of the first adjustments we make is not physical; it's mental. It's a transition from "What do I have?" and "Who can help me?" to "What can I do, what can I be, how else can I feel?" Instead of saying, "I see you can raise your arm only this high," I say, "Look how high you can raise your arm. That's where we're starting from, and that's what we are going to work with. Now what can you do?" My work is about empowering patients and then giving them the tools to help themselves.

Notice that curiosity is the fuel of the adaptation process. It's what leads us to ask, "What's wrong with me and how can I fix it?" or "I feel good, but how could I feel even better?" and then compels us to find out the answers. So rather than thinking of pain as something happening to you, you should see it as an opportunity to understand yourself better, to train your body for positive growth.

RESILIENCE

As I mentioned in my dancing analogy, active adaptation is self-reinforcing. The more we do it, the better we get at it. Over time, we learn how to feel the difference between "good pain" (which we can recover from) and "bad pain" (which might lead to serious injury or be the sign of a major problem). Then quite consciously and deliberately we can embrace and even introduce stress, welcoming the "good pain" that comes along with it, because we know we will be able to work through it. With each recurrence of that same stress, the body responds more and more effectively and efficiently, thanks in large part to our endogenous cannabinoid system (which we'll talk about in detail later). Our default becomes, incrementally, healthier and stronger. We improve our ability to deal with and bounce back from future stressors or stress more generally. We become more resilient. For example, surfers and swimmers mimic the breathing techniques of free divers, which can feel really uncomfortable, to improve their ability to hold their breath when they have to (a strategy introduced to me by Jessie Salas). Firefighters work through practice burns to gain tolerance to smoke and heat. The process doesn't need to be as extreme or intense as that; rather, think of it more like microdosing stress.

Still, stressing the body even mildly to overcome stress might sound counterintuitive. But the idea is to demystify the experience of stress, to make it more familiar and thus manageable.

Meanwhile, consider the alternative. If we avoid pain and stress, we give them power over us. We become afraid of the consequences because we haven't gone through them. Chemically speaking, giving in to fear of pain becomes a bad habit; in response to fear of pain, our body produces cortisol, and that becomes a pattern—cortisol for anticipated pain rather than actual pain. Consider weight training. If you take a break of some weeks or months and try to jump right back in again with the weight you were using earlier, the stress of that first lift is going to feel difficult; a 25-pound weight might feel like a 40-pound weight. That's because you haven't experienced that particular stress for a while, and our bodies depend on repetition in order to adapt.

Comedian Rodney Dangerfield often moaned loudly about "the heaviness," which was his hypochondriacal, depressive, overwhelming *fear* of something bad happening rather than of something bad actually happening. "Other people wake up in the morning, 'A new day! Ah, up and at 'em!' I wake up, the heaviness is waiting for me. Sometimes I even talk to it. I say, [adopts cheerful voice] 'Hi, heaviness!' and the heaviness looks back at me [in an ominous growl]: 'Today you're gonna get it good. You'll be drinking early today.'"

As bleak as Dangerfield's experience was, he was onto something that we all grapple with, in that liminal space between thought and behavior, mind and body, imagined and experienced. If we don't let ourselves go through stress, thus finding a way to adapt to that stress, the effort of pushing it aside or avoiding it will cause damage in all kinds of ways, both mental and physical. By muscling that stress away or by thinking we can completely avoid it, we augment the fear of its overwhelming us or of our having new stresses. Ultimately, that fear starts controlling our lives, limiting our potential in the most insidious of ways. As Sarno suggests, not engaging the stress of life head-on can even be the root of chronic pain.

THE TOOLS FOR HEALING

Curiosity fuels active adaptation, which brings about resilience. Resilience in turn encourages deeper curiosity and enables further active adaptation. This cycle of adaptation builds into generalized overall health. That's not to say you won't get injured or feel stress, but when it happens, you will be able to more effectively and efficiently deal with it and continue with a baseline of health. I am leading with this conceptual rationale because I see it as the core of any wellness regime that leads to true autonomy. Think of this rationale as your base of operation. Without it, you will never be able to break the "quick fix" mentality that dominates our reaction to pain. In order to adopt this new cycle of adaptation, I recommend three overarching protocols to incorporate into your daily life. Those protocols are:

1. Posture, Strength, and Breathing
2. Heat Therapy
3. Stimulation of the Endogenous Cannabinoid System

The general parameters of each of these three protocols are described below. Details will follow later in the book.

POSTURE, STRENGTH, AND BREATHING

One of the most essential things we can do to heal from chronic pain and manage physical stress is to learn how to recognize our poor movement patterns and positions, and then to correct them. That's what the posture, strength, and breathing exercises of Foundation Training are all about, and we'll explore them fully in the next chapter.

On the broadest level, this modality is about adapting actively when it comes to our physiology. The movement and breath work give us a physical understanding of how the muscle chains in our bodies are connected and the healthiest way we can occupy space. The goal is to demonstrate what your body feels like when its mass is disbursed among the most available muscle tissue possible. In that expansive position, we feel broad, tall, and light, because our body weight is distributed the way it's designed to be. We are taking up the most space we can, internally and externally, creating volume. In so doing, we relieve pressure from our joints, which is where we rest our weight when our posture is more complacent.

These expansive positions and movements work because when we train the body again and again to move correctly, it becomes second nature. Or to be more precise: it becomes first nature. We reteach our bodies what they were built to do in the first place: to move in efficient and healthy ways so we can stay strong and alive. To that end we must unlearn harmful movement habits and negative adaptations, allowing our bodies to return to primal patterns that have been disrupted by the stresses of modern life.

As you go through the postures and the breathing exercises that comprise Foundation Training, your body is stressed and undergoes subtle changes. Eventually, with enough repetition, that stress is something you adapt to in a positive way. And with each subsequent session, it takes increasing amounts of stress to provoke a reaction. In other words, through active adaptation, you're developing resilience.

People love to say, "Practice makes perfect," but nobody really explains why. Here's why: the more you train your body to do the right thing, to move the right way, the easier it is for your body to do it automatically. In fact, it becomes much harder to do it incorrectly.

HEAT

The second prong of my approach is heat—specifically, using the sauna to introduce positive stress in the form of perspiration, thus facilitating the body's lymphatic drainage system, which we'll talk about in chapter 3. As we train our body and mind to handle the stress of heat, we are training it to meet stress head-on in all areas of life.

Part of the skill of sauna is in accepting how your body responds, recognizing that your first sensations of anxiety do not mean you have to get out of the heat. That takes real mental training. You're learning about your stress response and your anxiety by confronting it directly and making the choice to stay in a stressful situation. The better you become at overriding your initial impulse to flee, the better you get at decision-making in general. You're testing your adaptivity. You're increasing your ability to maintain composure in moments of frustration, teaching yourself to make a positive decision in the face of adversity. We strengthen that sensation of resolve and perseverance necessary in all kinds of decisions concerning our health and life more generally. It's a discipline, and if you stay with it, pain relief seems easier, exercise seems easier, and emotional issues seem easier, too.

Heat therapy reinforces, and is reinforced by, the Foundation protocols of posture, strength training, and breathing. With heat, we're taking stress and using that energy and pushing it out through sweat. In Foundation Training, we use energy to actively contract muscles in order to support our body weight in and out of motion. They are both extreme metabolic expenditures, dependent on developing the skill of doing the exact same thing better next time.

STIMULATING THE ENDOCANNABINOID SYSTEM

The third tool of the protocol helps to explain why the first two are so effective. In all of us, there is a little-known system called the endocannabinoid system (ECS), which we will explore in much greater detail in later chapters.

Broadly speaking, the ECS is a master regulator for the whole body. It coordinates how our nervous system, immune system, hormonal system, and all of our organs respond to external and internal stress. It does that by registering and recording the stressful stimulus after it occurs, and then making our response to future exposures to that stimulus more efficient and effective. In short, it's how we adapt.

As I've said, life is all about adapting to stress, in one form or another, minute to minute. It can be the physical stress of intense exercise or the emotional stress of family vacation, a small stress like experiencing joint pain or meeting a stranger, or a bigger one like suffering an injury or falling in love. All we really are is an accumulation of our adaptations to the stresses in our lives so far.

Think about exercise. Adaptation comes because you're stressing your body to a point where it stimulates its need to change—a new response to pain, a new way to move or breathe—in order to make it through the end of the workout. That change occurs molecularly, at a chemical level. Most of us know that feeling at the end of a hard workout when you're thinking, *I'm almost there, almost there,* and there's this moment when you almost give up . . . but you don't. Every time you almost give up and don't, your body rewards you by creating a chemical that hits the button of pleasure—the endogenous cannabinoid anandamide. So your body now expects that pleasure the next time you push it toward stress. In addition, with experience, the pain and fear incrementally diminish as well. The next time you feel the exact same stress, it doesn't get that much easier, but you're a little more prepared for it. The hundredth time you encounter that same stress, it gets exponentially easier. And that's because you've repeated those minor stresses a little more frequently, so that your body is getting better at its response. That is your endogenous cannabinoid system, doing its job: making our everyday adaptations more and more efficient.

Because the endocannabinoid system is responsible for so many aspects of wellness, it is vital to keep this system functioning healthily. The two protocols I've already mentioned—posture, strength, and breathing exercises, as well as heat work—are key tools. More generally, taking conscious control of your exercise, diet, and overall lifestyle can nourish this system as well, as can the introduction of exogenous cannabinoids—cannabinoids from outside the body, derived from the plant cannabis.

With this broad-strokes picture in mind, let's now examine each of the three components in more detail. But first I want to return to Patti once more. When we left her, she was in so much pain she couldn't even pick up her beloved surfboard. But here she is after practicing some of the modalities we will be exploring in the next chapter and taking control of her life, a process that has taken years of concerted effort:

A lot of people want things handed to them, you know? They want the quick fix. They want it easy. But I think it's a lot of work, actually, to get yourself out of pain, and not everybody's in that kind of psychological or emotional or mental or spiritual place. In my experience, doing these poses and this breath work, really focusing on those skills, I noticed a difference pretty fast. I started feeling good about taking up space. For the first time, I felt like I deserve to be here in this body getting stronger. There's something super empowering about that. Like, to think, *I can fix myself, I don't need anybody else.* And with that belief, my body started to feel better, actually get stronger.

It's a beautiful thing, really, how the body affects the mind but the opposite is equally true. And best of all is the beautiful intelligence in the conversation between the two.

CHAPTER 2

Posture, Movement, Strength, and Breath

I've said this before, but it bears repeating: the way we move is wrong. All too often, our passive adaptations saddle us with unhealthy movement patterns, which create and reinforce long-term pain. When we respond to this pain with impatience and fear rather than curiosity, we become increasingly fragile and dependent on others.

In this chapter, we'll use posture, movement, strength, and breath work to turn all of those maladaptive behaviors around and learn how to treat and eliminate some of the most common forms of pain. We'll see how pain is an intersystemic, not just a local, issue. I introduce physical stress (through specific postures and movement) to help your body adapt productively, so that it becomes resilient to the common stresses of modern life. Deep down, at a neurological level, our bodies *want* to be efficient, because efficiency feels great and keeps us strong and healthy. Unlearning bad habits and passive adaptation—and reprogramming ourselves to move effectively—takes some work. But you're ready for it. And I promise you, it's the best way forward as a lifelong strategy for relief.

LISTEN TO THE WARNINGS

My first job is to try to engage my patients with their symptoms. If the pain they are feeling isn't the result of something structurally wrong (a ruptured ligament or torn muscle), then it's a symptom that their body is reacting to stress in an unhealthy way. These warning signs are opportunities for us to intervene, become curious, and choose a natural, healthy path instead, expanding our fundamental range of motion, improving our stress response, and encouraging active adaptation overall.

If all of a sudden your body is sending you a distress signal—an unusual new pain, trouble moving in a certain way not due to a specific injury—then I want you to go see other specialists before you even consider Foundation Training. Pain can be a symptom of an enormous range of conditions and diseases, and you have to rule out more serious things. If it is an acute injury or a pain that you are feeling for the first time, you need to go to the doctor or the clinic first; self-diagnosis of this kind of problem can screw you up pretty badly. But if you've been doing the same activities for years and you've had the same low-grade to high-grade pain that's just gotten worse over time—and you are fed up and want to change it—that's when Foundation Training comes into play. Typically, in these cases, the pain is being caused by something we're doing to ourselves. Foundation Training is also for people who just want to improve their somatosensation, to become more aware of how their body moves through space.

GOOD STRESS

Foundation Training shows us how to recognize poor movement patterns and correct them. But it's not an end unto itself. The movement, poses, and breath work all intentionally introduce stress as a way of training our bodies to adapt positively and thus become more resilient. As you learn to adapt to the techniques of Foundation Training, you also become more capable of handling life's other physical stressors, big and small: from picking up your baby or sitting on a plane to hiking up a mountain, stacking wood, planting a garden, or engaging in weight training.

While this section refers to FT poses and goes into some detail, please refer to the Gallery, in which a series of images of the basic postures are provided; to our certified instructors; to workout and pose tutorials at stream.foundationtraining.com; or to my two previous books, *Foundation* and *True to Form*, for more complete information.

WHAT'S IT ALL ABOUT?

The starting point for Foundation Training is the willingness to feel your body in new and unfamiliar ways. It's a series of body-weight exercises, meant to be done barefoot, that center your pelvis and expand your torso to the largest surface area it can sustain. We train those big, expansive muscles to know what it feels like when you're in a strong posture, and we practice that strong posture in various poses that strengthen and square the hips. We train the body to support its own weight.

I was taught in chiropractic school that correct posture is like a plumb line, where everything's lined up vertically. I now disagree with that wholeheartedly. I would argue that correct posture is about alignment, but it's also about standing or sitting in a way that engages the posterior muscle chain, the strongest chain in the body, so that your weight is distributed most efficiently. Let's try this. While standing, plant your feet parallel, about hip-width apart. Shift your hips back a little bit, away from your feet. Pull your neck back, stacking your head directly above your torso. Now consciously think about the relationship between your feet and hips and head. That line needs to be maintained no matter what position you're in, even seated. It is an active, powerful posture, which is what we want to be positively adapting toward.

Maintaining this healthy posture requires strength. It's important to remember that we are training for primary stability, which is active and keeps us aligned. Primary stability comes from muscles contracting against joints and muscles and tendons pulling joints into place. When injured, all of those can heal. By contrast, secondary stability is derived from ligaments, bones, and nonelastic connective tissue, which have minimal elasticity or active component and less capacity to heal. When these are injured, surgery is required. By strengthening the muscles of primary stability, we minimize our reliance on that less resilient secondary system.

Foundation Training focuses on two fundamental ranges of motion: hip hinging and rib cage movement (otherwise known as breathing). That's it. When you can perform those ranges of motion with legitimate strength, most other areas of the body fall

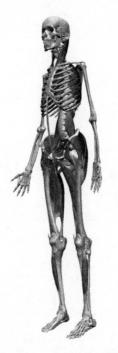

Do your best to make your feet as broad a surface area as you're able. Spread your toes and push your heels into the ground as you stand.

correctly in line. These exercises create more surface area around the spine and in the thoracic cavity (your chest), and the body is trained to have enough strength to maintain the space you've created.

The postures are exaggerated, which is intentional. Think of it as an overcorrection. Their purpose is to actively adapt your body so that when you fall back to a relaxed position—when you are walking down the street, sitting in a chair, brushing your teeth—you're reverting to a better overall baseline. Your default position, the way you move your body, is healthier—aligned and strong. It's all about repetition. Unlike weight lifting, Foundation Training doesn't require major recovery. It's frequency that does the work.

Underlying all the postures are the two central and complementary components of Foundation Training: anchoring and decompression. Let's take them one at a time:

ANCHORING

One of the major positions most of us have passively adapted to, both while we stand and sit, is to splay our feet out in a duckfooted position. This results in the external rotation of the femurs, away from the center of your body, which causes the glutes to shrink, so much so that they will adapt to their new truncated position. Adaptive shortening—or what should be called *maladaptive* shortening—occurs when a muscle, under the weight of gravity, under the force above it, simply lives in a shortened state so long that that's where it learns to operate from. Muscles are designed to go from elongated to shortened and back again, not from short to shorter. Anchoring is about adapting away from that position by emphasizing its opposite.

We are specifically anchoring our pelvis, which I consider the structural core of the body. People often think of the core as your abdominal muscles, but that's too far north. The pelvis is the body's true center of gravity. To be more precise, the center lies in the pubic symphysis, which is at the central spot where the two hemispheres/pieces of the pelvis meet.

Any muscle that directly connects to the pelvis is part of your core: hip flexors, glutes, hamstrings, iliaci (which run from the lowest rib to the top of the pelvis), and adductors (which, again, extend and wrap from the hip to the back of the femur, just in from where the glutes attach). These muscles are the puppet masters, the muscles that determine your body's center of gravity, and they're what we focus on when we anchor. You'll be feeling and working those muscles deliberately, in ways that you're probably not used to. I want you to lean into the newness of the sensation and know that it's going to feel strained at first. With practice, anchoring will become something you do unconsciously and without effort as your body begins to feel the benefits.

Anchoring squares the femurs forward by placing your feet parallel on the ground, maintaining pressure on their outer edges, then pulling the hips up and away from that, standing as tall as you can against that tension. It feels like the knees are squeezing toward each other and the joints in the big toe are squeezing toward each other. As the hips try to close toward center in the front—think of an ancient scroll closing—it creates more width at the back of the body.

Anchoring involves strengthening the muscles that start in the inner arch of the feet and run all the way up the insides of the groin to the pelvis, like a sling. Think of the arch of your left foot, the arch of your right foot, and the giant parabolic line of tension between them—like St. Louis' Gateway Arch between your legs. That big arch is being pulled upward from the center of both feet by the pelvis, providing tension up the leg, through the hamstrings, a series of smaller muscles around the knees, and then into the adductor muscles (the inner thigh). That upward lift, from the arches to the groin, the Gateway Arch, disperses the weight of the human body evenly—around the pubic symphysis, through every muscle that connects to the core. That's the strongest pull in the body—the downward-upward pull between the arches and the bottom of the pelvis.

Let's look at why the adductors are so important. Unlike the hamstrings, the adductor does not cross the knee joint; it inserts right *above* the knee joint. This helps to give it a much stronger

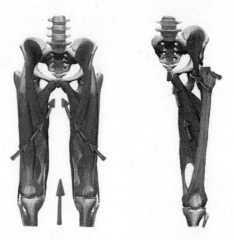

The upward arrows note the drive of force toward the pubic symphysis, or center of the pelvis. The adductor muscles attach bilaterally to the pubic symphysis.

pull on the femur toward the center of the body, without any interruption or influence from anything else. But just as important is *how* the adductor attaches to the femur that it pulls. In most other muscle-bone connections in the body, a relatively small surface area of muscle and bone are connected. But here, most of the adductor is connected to most of the femur. All the meat is glued to the bone. So when the muscle contracts, it is able to take the whole bone with it. That's a lot of power, and we're meant to use it. The adductor isn't just pulling the hips together; it's a key part of the activation of a whole chain of other muscles as well—all the way down to the bottom of the foot. When the adductors are in a shortened state and turned away from each other, it causes problems in the knees, hips, and lower back. By making sure they are in the proper position and strengthening them, we can both prevent and correct these issues.

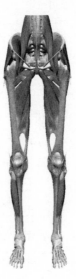

The muscles on the outer thigh depend on the muscles along the inner thigh in order to function healthily.

The better you anchor, the more your legs are working to support your entire body, the more secure your pelvis is and the more you can decompress your spine up and outward, away from that very strong platform.

TAKE A DEEP BREATH

Once you're anchored, you can decompress.

Decompression, through breath work, is about creating space around the twelve joints of the thoracic spine. Right along this spine is much of the autonomic nerve system, which controls the automatic decisions our body makes: function of internal organs, regulation of heart rate, digestion and respiration, sexual arousal, pupil dilation, and the fight-or-flight response. *Each of those things independently* can be impaired when the tissues here are compressed (recall how my digestive troubles were linked to my spinal injury). So the more room we can give that system, the healthier its tissues become.

Decompression happens from the pelvis all the way up to the top of the head, and it's all about creating width across the body, which creates internal space. Simply put, the Foundation Training mission is to reeducate the axial skeleton toward expansion. Think of it like an umbrella: the lower spine is the stem of the umbrella, which opens at the rib cage, up to the head.

The head is the very center of the umbrella, pulling upward as the sides of the umbrella expand. But just as an umbrella doesn't function well if half of it remains closed, you have to make sure you have a full expansion all the way around, which occurs primarily at the rib cage level. We are aiming for a big lift of the circumference of the rib cage and torso, creating more internal space.

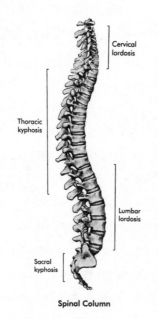

Cervical
lordosis

Thoracic
kyphosis

Lumbar
lordosis

Sacral
kyphosis

Spinal Column

The varied curves of a healthy spine.

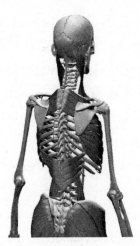

Note the serratus muscles, which connect the rib cage to the spinal column. And the anterior serratus, which connect the shoulder blade and the rib cage.

The way to initiate this is to lift the sternum. If the sternum is dropped, you're doing the opposite of decompression; you're rounding your shoulders forward, compressing and shrinking your internal surface area. The first cue I usually give is "Chest up!" Immediately, you are creating more space inside your body. Pause for a moment right now and notice whether your sternum is lifting forward and up or slumped down toward the back of your body.

In a healthy breath, the sternum lifts as a direct result of the increase width of the rib cage. Take a deep breath and really feel how your sternum lifts forward as your rib cage expands in all directions. Manipulating the back of the rib cage, in particular, has an enormous physical and emotional impact. The psoas muscle, which connects the spine to the femur, is also connected (through fascia and ligaments) to the diaphragm. The diaphragm controls our breath, and by extension affects our emotional state. Think about when you are nervous. You take shallow, rapid breaths. When you are relaxed, you take slow, deep, expansive breaths. A tight psoas is a signal to our body that we are in danger. That fight-or-flight response has been activated. Learning how to breathe in a way that decompresses and expands this vital area of the body relaxes and stretches the psoas. It requires reeducating the upper skeleton, using decompression breathing to teach the psoas to actively adapt to a healthier position.

It's important to underline which muscles we're not engaging, too. For far too long, the lower spine and the abdominal area have been the center of people's rehabilitative motions—crunches at the gym, spinal twists in yoga. But the fact is, the lower spine is really not designed to move that much. It just needs to be stable, which means the lower back is strong enough to communicate with all the other muscles in the body and not be dominated by them. Overworking the abs can in fact work against this by weakening the back muscles that move and support the spine.

Where we're really built to move, the truly muscular part of our upper body, is well above the lower spine—at the thoracic cage and shoulders. Here, movement occurs with minimal focal points of pressure. It is expansion in all directions. It's that umbrella opening. This torso expansion is difficult for everyone at first, and most of my patients have a hard time locating the muscles involved when we first start working together. We simply aren't used to feeling the back side of our bodies expand. That's unpracticed somatosensation.

What does a deep, healthy active breath look like? Shoulders wide and head lifting. Your lats (upper back muscles) strong, fully engaged and firing. Inside, fully expanded lungs and a contraction of the diaphragm that pushes the liver and other organs down and the ribs wider and away from each other.

Decompression breathing expands the torso and lifts the rib cage away from the lower torso, creating space for all those vital organs, visceral tissues, and dense confluences of nerves in the upper body. By increasing their surface area, you increase the efficacy of all of these internal systems, including the nervous system and the lymphatic system. With more space, bodily processes become healthier and more efficient.

THE MOST COMMON FORMS OF PAIN

The principles of anchoring and decompression can be used to effectively prevent and treat most common ailments. In this section, we'll explore each of those ailments in detail, from symptoms to treatments to outcomes.

As we've discussed, pain is the most common way the body

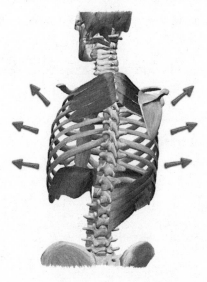

The collective effort of decompression breathing is axial expansion toward the back edges, sides, and front of the torso.

signals that something is wrong and that we need to start paying attention. Our attention often comes in the form of resistance and dread—especially when pain is involved. But as I keep saying, getting curious sets you more solidly on a path to healing than fear. While the specifics in the following stories vary—a professional stand-up paddleboarder with a debilitating neck injury, a surfer with spondylolisthesis so bad he couldn't pick up his child, a firefighter with sciatica—you'll start to see a pattern of adaptation and healing across the spectrum of patients. In each instance, the patient's educated efforts and discipline allowed healing to occur without invasive techniques.

Because of the interconnected or systems-based ways our bodies function, symptoms are almost always interwoven. If you have spondylolisthesis (one vertebra slipping onto the bone below it), often one of your symptoms will be sciatica (pain from your lower back into your hips, butt, and legs), as well as centralized low back pain and sometimes front hip pain. If you have scoliosis (sideways curvature of the spine), you're likely to have sciatica, and frequently carpal tunnel or thoracic outlet syndrome (numbness and tingling in the hand and arm). It's still useful to talk about these issues one at a time so that we can learn how they are interrelated and come up with the best plan to treat them.

BELOW THE BELT

Sciatica: The Root of the Problem

Matt, a respected but traditional chiropractor, noticed that he was having difficulty lifting the front of his right foot. He thought he'd just pulled a muscle and that it would get better with rest. It didn't. Instead, his foot and ankle felt increasingly weak, and it took a lot of effort not to drag his toe on the ground when he walked. Climbing stairs became very difficult, and soon he was feeling a numbness in his ankle.

These symptoms alarmed Matt. He knew this to be a condition called foot drop or drop foot, and its most serious causes could be stroke, multiple sclerosis (MS), or even amyotrophic lateral sclerosis (ALS). Traditional treatments include shoe inserts, physical therapy, and leg braces, and if there is no improvement, a surgery that fuses the ankle and foot bones. After visiting a fellow chiropractor and an acupuncturist and being told by a neurologist that nothing was wrong with his MRI, Matt found his way to me.

When most doctors address foot drop, they are focused on the peroneal nerve, which runs from the back of the knee to the shin. It's true that the nerve is fairly close to the surface of the skin and can therefore sometimes be injured, but that's not the underlying issue. Which means traditional treatments—like applying a splint or strengthening the foot and ankle—are not going to do anything for long-term healing.

When Matt came to me, he was surprised at my response. In most cases, I told him, foot drop doesn't have anything to do with the foot itself, or even with the knee. We had a chiropractor-to-chiropractor conversation where I got to fire up my thrillingly multi-colored anatomy app program (Visible Body) with someone who really appreciated it. I pointed to a muscle called the tibialis anterior, which stretches from the bottom of the foot to the shin and controls the movement of the top outer bones of the foot. It's this muscle that allows us to flex the foot up and back.

Together, Matt and I traced the peroneal nerve, which is connected to the tibialis anterior, up the shin to the knee, where it is revealed to be a branch of a much larger nerve coming down the leg: the sciatic nerve. We kept following the sciatic nerve up into the pelvis.

And that's where the true cause of foot drop lies: the root of the sciatic nerve, which is at the sacroiliac (SI) joint. The SI joint connects the sacrum (the large wedge-shaped vertebra at the end of the spine that forms the solid base of the spinal column) with the bones of the pelvis. In fact, foot drop is just one of a host of symptoms that all relate to this same spot: a condition collectively known as sciatica pain that specifically originates from the sciatic nerve. Your doctor might also call it lumbar radiculopathy or radicular pain.

Symptoms of sciatica can range from a dull ache or constant burning to shooting pain, numbness, tingling, a feeling like an electric shock, or general intermittent weakness. These feelings can occur anywhere along the sciatic nerve, from the lower back and the butt down the front or back of your thigh to your calf and foot.

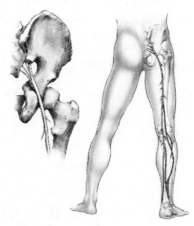

The long sciatic nerve pathway.

The symptoms might worsen when you're in different positions—sitting, trying to stand up, bending the spine forward, twisting the spine, or lying down. It's not uncommon for patients to live with this slowly worsening pain for decades, untreated.

Sciatica can be caused by disc degeneration (including bulges and herniations), spinal arthritis, pregnancy, a muscle spasm, a pinched nerve, and very rarely tumors, blood clots, or a severe injury to the sciatic nerve itself. But far more often, it is caused simply by moving your hip and/or pelvis the wrong way. If you squeeze your butt muscles, they contract, the tissue gets shorter, and the femurs rotate away from each other. The hips open in the front and close up in back, leveraging the sacroiliac joints (which connect your pelvis and lower spine). That's the duckfooted position I mentioned earlier. Also, recall that when you sit all the time, the glutes shrink and weaken under the weight of gravity.

Those weakened and shortened glute muscles create compression between the pelvis and the lower spine. All of that compression encroaches upon the sciatic nerve and limits its function. It can be felt in the form of nerve pain running down the leg. In Matt's case, the compression literally prevented the sciatic nerve from transmitting a signal, via the peroneal nerve, to the tibialis anterior below it—resulting in foot drop. But, more globally, that compression also impacts the function of everything else around it: the digestive tissue (colon) that is directly in front of the lumbar spine and the lymphatic tissue present in the area.

Some palliative measures that are prescribed for sciatica I'm fine with: ice or heat, exercise, massage, and acupuncture. Others are bad news: pain relievers and muscle relaxants, occasionally an epidural steroid injection. Sciatic symptoms can be placated and muffled forever, but until they are addressed at the source, there's likely no lasting improvement.

Traditionally, doctors have treated sciatica at a very mechanical level, at the point of occurrence: at the back of the hips, in the behind-the-buttocks tissue, down the leg into these peripheral branches of the nerve. Because it's seen as a "back of the body" issue, treatment is focused on the external rotators of the hip, the muscles that lever the leg out.

But these treatments presume a "front-to-back" relationship between the body's muscles. In fact, it's an upward, spiraling, twisting relationship. The glutes (again, the muscles that run along the body's outside edges, extending and wrapping from pelvis all the way down to the back of the thigh) are impacted by the adductors (muscles that run along on the body's inner edges, extending and wrapping from the hip to the back of the femur, just in from where the glutes attach). This relationship delivers a focal point of pressure to the back edges of the hips, which ultimately alters everything happening in the hip socket.

The hip socket is where sciatica starts. Like many sciatic patients, Matt was told by a well-meaning physical therapist to strengthen his glutes with external rotation, but that only made things worse. In fact, it's not the glutes that need attention, but the muscles that challenge the glutes—namely the adductor longus (one of the adductors that runs along the thigh) and the iliacus (which flexes the thigh at the hip). If that centralizing pull from the adductors is not strong and even, it can do more than cause sciatica. As we'll see below, it creates everything from sacroiliac joint dysfunction, plantar fasciitis, scoliosis, and numerous other symptoms that you would never think originate in the pelvis.

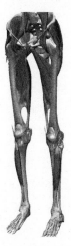

Here we see the tibialis anterior along the shin, adductors along the inner femur, and the gluteal, iliacus, and psoas combination lining the hip joints.

The best way to strengthen the endurance of the adductors is through the practice of anchoring. The goal is to secure and tighten these muscles so that they are actively pulling *away* from the sciatic nerve. The key is internal rotation, creating space by actively closing the gate in front of the body, which then opens up the back of the body. That space is required for healthy nerve flow to the tibialis anterior. Once the nerve flow is healthy, the muscles will receive the signal to contract.

It took no time at all for Matt to learn to anchor. He strengthened his adductors, the pain ebbed right away, and before he knew it, his foot was flexing as it was supposed to. Unlike any other treatment for sciatica that I know of, anchoring solves the problem for good. This is what we mean by actively adapting. By stressing the correct muscles in unfamiliar ways, we alter our posture and movement patterns to a healthier default.

Before we start moving up the body, I want to address two

incredibly common symptoms that occur below the pelvis: plantar fasciitis and knee pain. Just like sciatica, both signal a weakness or misalignment in the arch of tension that helps distribute our body weight in an even and efficient manner.

Plantar Fasciitis

Plantar fasciitis is one of the most common causes of heel pain. It involves inflammation of a thick band of tissue that runs across the bottom of your foot and connects your heel bone to your toes. This pain traditionally plagues runners, but everyone over the age of forty is susceptible to it.

Both the anterior tibialis muscle (on the outside of the lower leg) and the posterior tibialis muscle (in the rear of the lower leg) insert into the medial arch of the foot, creating a sling that lifts the top of the foot toward the pubic symphysis. Conventional treatment focuses on the foot itself: stretching the tendons, injecting steroids to reduce the swelling.

But think of the leg as a whip. The strongest part of the whip happens at the hip joint; the crack of the whip occurs at the foot. In plantar fasciitis, there is too much muscle tension at the low end of the whip and not enough range of motion in the hips. When hip mobility is limited, it puts more pressure on the ankle and foot. All that tension—which in a healthy body is shared by the more powerful muscles of the hip, groin, and hamstrings—is located in the foot, which isolates the work the foot has to perform. If we don't properly engage the hips to help distribute the tension, the foot is overtaxed, causing inflammation and pain.

For people suffering from plantar fasciitis, I recommend the wide leg founder (see the Gallery), paying particular attention to the three points of contact between the foot and the ground. The toes should be lifted away from the ground and spreading away from each other. The arches of the feet should be pulling up away from the floor, into the center of gravity (the pubic symphysis). I also recommend integrated hinges (see the Gallery), keeping the feet in the position described above. Hinges will help distribute the excess tension in the arches of the feet to the more powerful muscles of the hips.

Knee Pain: Jessie's Story

Many of my patients suffer from knee pain, and it is often the reason people stop leading active lives. In his earlier career, Jessie Salas was a firefighter for the city of Orlando, in a special operations unit. On top of that physically demanding job, Jessie strength-trained on the side, like a lot of people on the force, and he practiced Brazilian jiujitsu. When he tore a medial collateral ligament, or MCL (the band of tissue on the inside of your knee that connects your thigh bone to the bone of your lower leg), I offered my services. At that time, I was still mostly working with people with lower back pain, so I had to convince Jessie that I could help him. After a couple of exercises, he recalls:

> What I realized right away is that engaging the muscles around my knee brought stability and support. We began essentially retraining how my knee functioned. It could be strong and supported by leveraging the right muscles, instead of just depending on the MCL, which was pretty much all I was relying on for support.

Jessie's knee had taken a direct hit. His MCL was torn, but by strengthening his auxiliary muscles, he got back his strength and support, which allowed the ecosystem around the MCL injury the time to heal on its own. We worked to strengthen his primary mode of stability to give his secondary mode time to recover. No surgery was involved. Now, the MCL itself may never fully heal, but because he strengthened what's around that tissue, the knee is no longer unstable. There's a preventative purpose to this work, too; Jessie firmly believes that if he'd had these tools earlier, he would never have had this injury in the first place.

When no structural issue like Jessie's torn MCL is involved, knee pain is most often actually caused by something happening at the ankles or the hips. The reason for this is that weakness above or below the knee signals the knee to make up for those weaknesses, adding extra stress to the joint that already has plenty to do. So when my patients experience knee pain, the first thing I do is teach them how to use their feet correctly. Anchoring and activating that long arch of muscles results in a stable leg up the ankle, through the knee, and up to the hip.

For additional stability, I often recommend a hip hinge— showing patients that the knee isn't supposed to be the first thing to bend. Rather, the hips must get out of the way and *then* the knees can bend. That's how the body moves most efficiently.

If you are too weak to maintain a proper arch of tension to anchor you firmly and correctly to the ground, your knees are going to bear the brunt of that. Foundation Training instructors often share stories of patients who didn't get the recommended meniscus or ACL, PCL, or LCL surgery. Instead, they strengthened their hamstrings, glutes, and adductors in the right way, eradicating pain or stability issues. In so doing, they buttressed the knee joint and adjusted their movement patterns to keep it secure.

At first Jessie thought the postures we were doing were just delaying some inevitable surgery. But only a couple of weeks after his tear, he was up and surfing comfortably. Jessie was such a convert that he ended up leaving his job as a firefighter and becoming a Foundation trainer alongside me. Here's what he has to say about the work we do to shift the focus from localized concerns ("my knee hurts!") to the awareness that pain is usually the symptom of a larger mechanical problem:

> We're teaching people how to recruit more muscles, instead of just overtaxing the ones they consistently rely on. As we go through life, we develop imbalances. And Foundation work very quickly targets those imbalances. You end up strengthening and leveraging all the muscles involved in healthy movement.

ABOVE THE BELT

Now let's move up the body. Just as important as what's below our center of gravity at the pelvis is what's above. Remember the body's most important pull? It's the adductors, lifting the bottom of the pelvis and creating an arch of tension that brings the feet and the hips toward each other. That arch of tension is complemented by what's going on right above the pelvis: the upward lift and expansion of the thoracic cage (rib cage). These two forces snap our centers into place.

To explore this upper-lower relationship, let's look at a common condition where it really comes into play: scoliosis. Our best possible guide here is Josh Holland, a trainer whom I met while we were both working with the same client. Here's Josh's story:

Scoliosis: Josh Holland

I was in high school, in Oklahoma. One day a chiropractor happened to be visiting our school, and I told him I always had this nagging pain in my back. It wasn't debilitating in any way, because I was one of our star athletes. He had me touch my toes, and looked at my back and went, "It looks fine, but . . ."—he didn't want to scare me—"Why don't you come to my office when you get some time?" His office was walking distance from my house. He took a bunch of X-rays and told me I had scoliosis. When he showed me the curvature in my spine, he said, "Imagine if we could either slow down the progression of the curvature or slowly take out some of that curvature. Imagine how much taller you would be." I was a serious basketball player and hoping to get recruited for college. He gave me exercises to do every day and manipulated my spine, and I did start to feel a little better, but I think it was more the mental, the placebo effect of it.

When I became a trainer, I wanted to fix my back because I was tired of feeling weak, and also a lot of the people I was working with at the time had low back pain and I wanted to help them. I was very quick to identify when someone else had scoliosis. I was doing some fitness modeling at the time, and I remember I did a test shoot for *Men's*

Health magazine. Everything was fine from the front and from the side, but when the photographer started taking pictures of my back, he said, "Hey, stand up straight for me." In my brain I'm like, "I am." But I learned to manipulate myself. I'd look at my ribs and shift myself into a position that allowed me to be straighter.

It worked, but just temporarily. I still experienced weakness, and I still didn't have a long-term treatment plan that addressed my back issues.

Scoliosis is simply a curvature of the spine. We all know that the spine curves front to back. Scoliosis is a lateral curvature of the spine, when it kinks left or right. Congenital or structural scoliosis (a condition you're born with) is extremely rare and hard to change. In all but extreme cases, we might be able to help you improve your quality of life up to 40 or 50 percent—still a better outcome than any surgery.

Then there's the much more common type: functional scoliosis, which is a learned pattern. This, too, is a very hard fix, and I understand and empathize with people who are forced to face it. But it is possible, as we'll see in a minute.

Left untreated or improperly treated, scoliosis can cause a wide swath of other problems in the body. Because those spinal kinks occur at nerve junctures and at nerve plexuses (branching networks of intersecting nerves), even mild scoliosis can cause nerve damage, numbness, and leg pain. More severe cases throw the knees and hips off balance, leaving you prone to falls and unable to walk for very long.

Then there are the effects on the body's organs. A scoliotic spine curvature can have a direct impact on organs like the liver, the spleen, the pancreas, and digestive organs, and it can compress the space around them. It can limit lung volume, alter heart rate, and in extreme cases, impact the prostate. One of my scoliosis patients has chronic hepatitis—not from disease itself, but from chronic inflammation of the liver. Her spine had rotated into the liver, and every time she moved, it pushed into that organ, which inflamed it over and over.

Scoliosis is usually treated directly at the spine, just like Josh's chiropractor did. Exercises and physical therapy can certainly help, but only temporarily and incompletely. Braces are used for childhood scoliosis, but they tend to make the muscles weaker, which only compounds the problem. All too often, people with chronic scoliosis turn to quick fixes like painkillers or epidural steroid injections (remember my patient Patti Sheaff from chapter 1). Then of course there's back surgery (that is to say, fusion), and I think you know by now how I feel about that. A traditional chiropractic treatment for scoliosis would be to align the spine, which will indeed help the nerve and tissues touched and influenced by the curvature. But the spine, just like any other part of the body, doesn't exist in a vacuum. We need to train the muscles that support it.

I encouraged Josh to think about and feel out the connections in his body. As he discovered, the true point of origin for scoliosis is not the spine, but rather the spine's platform: the pelvis. Here's how:

In our natural state, everything is pulling upward in the body. Our hips, which support the spine, are pulling up, and our head is pulling up away from it. But when we lose that upward-pulling battle against gravity, our weight drops and creates these compression points below. In scoliosis, the pelvic girdle (where the spine sits at the sacrum) is inadequately stabilized from weakness in the legs below. As a result, it cantilevers or tilts a few degrees left or right at an incline. That tilt starts a pitch that the spine follows, and now there's weight on top of that pitch. You know those portable cups that people take camping, the ones that look like a flat disc until you spin it up, locking it securely into place? That's a healthy spine. In scoliosis, the movement occurs in the opposite direction, and the spine spirals down, collapsing on itself.

Our vertebrae move in what's called coupled motion. When the spine flexes, it doesn't just move back and forth, it also rotates. But in scoliosis, that mechanism is weakened, and under the weight of gravity, the spine rotates and collapses down on itself. Think of an old biplane if the engine cuts out. It begins to spiral downward. The center of the curve becomes the primary folding point, so that's where you'll see the most drastic and dramatic change.

While scoliosis initiates below the pelvis, it continues the reaction of the spine and the rib cage above it. And that's where we'll treat it. What we're after—with scoliosis and all the other symptoms and forms of pain in this section—is decompression.

When Josh started employing the intentional stress of decompression breathing, he noticed a difference pretty quickly. And the more he worked, the bigger and more long-lasting the difference got. Through regular decompression breathing, he learned to actively manipulate his spine, build strength around it, increase the space limited by its curve. With much work, he was able to engage the elastic potential of his upper spine, teaching the muscles that support it to find their former length so that they moved beyond their maladaptive shortened state.

Pretty soon, Josh was actually straightening the curve and

holding it straight! Adapting actively, he pushed his body to a point of extreme stress, out of its comfort zone, so that after every session, his return to "normal" or balance was a little bit closer to straight. It has been a ton of hard, sweaty work, a process of constant tug-of-war, more active awareness of where he is pulling, where he is expanding. He continues to make thrilling progress.

Carpal Tunnel Syndrome: The Whip

Another common symptom that brings people to my door is carpal tunnel syndrome, which all too many who type or use a computer mouse are acquainted with. That kind of repetitive motion creates compression of the median nerve, which runs the length of your arm, through the narrow carpal tunnel at the wrist, and into your hand. The syndrome usually presents as pain, numbness, or weakness in the wrist and hands.

Once again, the traditional treatment for this pervasive issue focuses too much on the point of pain. Stretching, icing, wrist braces—I'm not against any of those things, but just like plantar fasciitis, if you don't see how the pain fits into the bigger picture, you're not going to find lasting relief. As always, there is a surgical solution offered for severe cases, which involves cutting the ligament that sits on top of the carpal tunnel, to relieve pressure on the median nerve. To be blunt, I have never met a single person who was glad they'd had that surgery. Eventually, they will work with someone like me, learning to use their arm in a way that alleviates their pain.

But to do that right, you must understand the bigger picture.

Remember how I said the leg was like a whip, with the most powerful part of it being the hip joint? Think of the arm in much the same way. The most powerful part is not the hand, not the arm, but the muscle that connects the upper arm to the spine and hip: the latissimus dorsi muscle, which covers the width of the middle and lower back and is the largest muscle in the upper body. From our lats, power and tension are driven down the arm to the hand.

So let's follow the whip from the hand backward up the arm to the latissimus dorsi. While we're at it, let's trace the median nerve backward through the carpal tunnel up the arm to its root, between the neck and the shoulder, at a very important grouping of nerves called the brachial plexus. Every sensation and motor impulse in the chest, shoulder, arm, forearm, and hand, every strength and weakness in these places: it comes through nerves (like the median nerve) that originate in the brachial plexus.

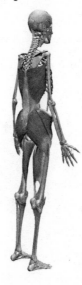

Here we see the power centers of the upper and lower limbs: the latissimus dorsi below the shoulder girdle and the gluteals behind the hip complex. The conventional core muscles live within and between these two powerful places.

But as we saw with sciatica, the root of the problem isn't in the nerve; it's in the muscles surrounding them. Specifically, the lats. With carpal tunnel, there is likely a weakness of and miscommunication between the lats, the shoulder joint, and the cervical-thoracic joints (which connect the spine's vertebrae). When those areas (the powerful end of the whip) are weak, they compress the brachial plexus, which results in nerve pain all the way down the median nerve to the fingers. So just paying attention to the wrist or hand (the end of the whip) is not going to provide long-term relief.

Foundation Training's solution to carpal tunnel syndrome is to directly address the compression on the brachial plexus. When you recruit the lat muscles, they pull the shoulders apart, creating space at the neck and relieving the pressure. An accurate lat contraction is one of the most important things the body can learn, and it is the most sustainable long-term fix for carpal tunnel. We teach accurate lat contractions in every single one of our exercises. They're quite a workout, and that's on purpose: with each contraction, with each expansive breath, we're actively stressing the muscle in an exagger-

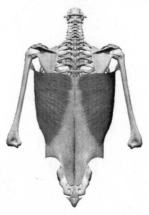

Just imagine a couple heavy suitcases being carried and you can see and feel the latissimus dorsi muscles in action.

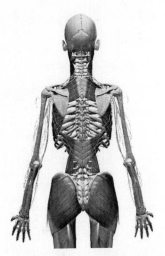

The brachial plexus and the other nerve confluences within the body are deserving of your attention and study.

ated way so that its return to normal gives the tissue at the brachial plexus more space. The healthier we can get that tissue, the better chance we have of creating strength and range of motion. The whole whip is now more resilient and powerful, all the way to the fingertips.

Frozen Shoulder

I want to briefly mention another condition that occurs when the thoracic cage is out of balance and that can be improved via correct engagement of the lats. Anyone over the age of fifty has a tendency to lose a substantial amount of range of motion in the shoulder joints if they don't pay attention. The extreme version of this is called frozen shoulder (adhesive capsulitis), when the shoulder is just stuck. People spend thousands of dollars getting their shoulder treated and treated and treated, and oftentimes opt for different release surgeries. But those surgeries take you to such a limited place, severely curtailing future movement and flexibility.

The way I teach shoulder health is by stabilizing the muscles and ligaments behind and below it. The lat muscle protects the bottom of the shoulder, pulling it back and into the shoulder joint. But that's not the same as retracting your shoulder blades, which pulls the shoulders together behind you. To know if you are doing it correctly, pay attention to the movement of your shoulder blades (you'll need a mirror or a partner): when you move your arm in any direction, your shoulder blade should move in the same direction, but about a third as much. So if my shoulder moves six inches, my shoulder blade should move approximately two inches in the same direction. Three to one.

When your shoulder blade and your rib cage stop communicating well, your shoulder blade gets very sticky. And that comes down to the serratus muscles, which stabilize the shoulder blade against the rib cage. If we are breathing well, our ribs should be expanding, and the shoulder blade should be expanding along with it. In a healthy body, that is maintained. In an unhealthy pattern, the belly moves too much when you breathe, almost exclusively, and the rib cage hardly moves at all: the shoulder motion is not perpetuated with the breath. The first innocent bystander of that poor breathing pattern is the shoulder complex and the neck. As the rib cage collapses and drops instead of expanding, the shoulders and neck converge forward, which puts pressure on the discs and therefore the brachial plexus. To combat that maladaptive pressure, we need to expand the rib cage, to give the shoulders and serratus muscles—and the shoulder blades—a more stable platform. From that platform, shoulder movement starts to improve very quickly, and your body actively adapts to that healthier breath pattern and movement. A fully expanding rib cage and a stable pelvic base are the real key to long-term healing of frozen shoulder.

Neck and Shoulder Pain: Seychelle's Story

Now that we know the brachial plexus is a group of nerves that runs from the shoulder up through the neck, it's no surprise that its compression can also cause neck pain. I want to introduce you to another person, someone whose neck pain was so severe it compromised not only her well-being but also her livelihood. Seychelle Webster is a professional stand-up paddleboarder. Relatively new to the sport, she quickly became one of the world's most elite competitors. She was used to pain, and thought it came with the job of being a high-performance athlete. Her body was ridiculously strong and conditioned, but one day, as Sychelle describes it, she woke up, tried to stretch, and felt so much pain that she started to panic. "I went to urgent care. I was like, 'I'm fucked up, I need help.' It was a serious amount of pain that I'd never experienced before. My neck was in excruciating pain, and it radiated all down my arm and into my hand, and my fingers were numb."

Seychelle, who doesn't take pain medication and prides herself on a non-Western approach to health, was terrified to get an MRI, because she feared that would lead to the suggestion of a surgical intervention. After almost two weeks of not sleeping because the pain was so great, she decided to see a neurosurgeon, who, after studying her diagnostic images, recommended immediate surgery. He wanted to perform a spinal fusion from C5 to C7—right where the brachial plexus is located. Other doctors proposed different options, but these all involved some sort of neck surgery, which would have put Seychelle out of commission for months and have seriously jeopardized her career.

Determined to find an alternative before she went under the knife, Seychelle reached out to her fans on social media for advice. Through them, she heard about Foundation Training and decided to give it a try. What she learned was that she needed to undo a lifetime of poor movement patterns.

A lot of what I had to learn in my recovery was how out of balance I was. My body was so strong, but it had been built up incorrectly. And I had reached the point where I couldn't push anymore, I was in too much pain. My main imbalance that led to severe neck pain was using my traps over my lats. In order to heal, I had to learn how to engage lats over traps.

In the same way that lat muscles are key to solving shoulder and wrist issues, they are also essential in addressing neck pain. Over-developing her traps (the large muscle in the upper back) and underutilizing her lats (the muscle in the lower and middle back) had thrown Seychelle's body completely out of balance. She was strong enough to overcompensate . . . until she wasn't. By engaging her lats and making sure her head and neck were in the correct balanced position, she found immediate pain relief.

But Seychelle also realized she had more changes to make.

I had to retrain myself. My whole technique was based on getting power from my upper body, when really I should have been getting power from my hips. Paddling is a full body movement, so I had to learn how to paddle without using my shoulders and my neck. I taught myself how to totally relax in the shoulders and to really just use my lower body.

Her new technique vastly improved her performance.

Recovering from this injury and retraining and rebalancing my body made me even faster. I had suffered this traumatic injury and thought, *That's it, I'm done, it's over*. And yet by the summer I became world champion. Foundation Training became my fifteen-minute warm-up, just breathing and reminding my body the right way to move. I gained a lot more body awareness than I previously had. It's not like there's just one exact right or wrong way to do a movement—your body could be built a different way. But I do think that there is a biomechanically optimized way to do it. Especially when you've had a severe injury, you have to do it that way to heal.

It wasn't just rethinking her stroke that helped Seychelle, it was rethinking how she moved through everyday life. Being aware of which muscles should be firing, how her body should be positioned, and actively adapting to these new, healthier patterns made all the difference. And not only did Seychelle heal herself, she went on to win the 2019 AAP Stand Up Paddling World Championship.

That final point above is crucial. Healing continues to happen even when you are not pushing yourself at a sport. It happens every single day. Seychelle also coaches paddleboarding, and when her clients feel pain, they always blame the sport. She's quick to point out that oftentimes paddleboarding itself is not causing the issue.

> When they have injuries or pain, I always say, "That's not just from your paddling, that's from what you're doing after you're paddling." I'm like, "We can adjust your stroke, but if you're just gonna go sit slumped at your computer all day after that, you know, I can't help you." But I guess I was the same way until my body broke down.

THE WHOLE BODY

I want to touch on a few other common symptoms, whose proper treatment involves everything we just learned: addressing the arc of tension in the lower half of the body and engaging the expansive upward lift of the thoracic cage.

Spondylolisthesis: Erik's Story

Spondylolisthesis (shortened to "spondy" by everyone, for obvious reasons) is a condition where one of the lower vertebrae slips forward, hitting the bone beneath it. It can be extremely painful, and given what we know about how the spine is supposed to twist and flex upwards, it causes issues that radiate up and down the body. Erik Antonson, who has one of the severest cases of spondy I have seen, first started noticing his back issues when he moved to Costa Rica and his life changed in a couple of big ways.

I went from surfing a couple hours a few times a week to surfing six hours a day. That amount of prone paddling really started aggravating my back. But it wasn't terrible until we had our daughter, Kemper. I would walk around and hold her, which I loved, but after about fifteen, twenty minutes, I'd be in so much pain. Just in that front-loading weight position, my feet would go numb. And at around that point, I started realizing I had a pretty big problem.

After getting two MRIs, which showed that the spondy was getting worse, Erik went the chiropractic route for a while.

It wasn't real relief and I couldn't do it myself, and living in Costa Rica, you were six hours from someone who could do it. I mean, I would drive to San Jose every once in a while, it would get so bad, so I could get that relief for a few days. And then I started thinking more about spinal fusion.

But after the same agonizing, terrified debate about surgery that Seychelle had gone through, Erik, too, sought out a different path.

By the time I met him, my thinking on spondy had really been evolving. In chiropractic school, we were taught to fix spondy with flexion movements to increase mobility. But that never made any sense to me. Why would you try to add movement to an unstable spine?

You don't stabilize a spondy at the vertebrae level. Rather, as I came to see with Erik and my other spondy patients, you work with what's around the vertebrae: the muscles. Specifically, you engage the adductor muscles and that downward vector of force, and you lift and expand the thoracic cage above it. Like a Chinese finger trap that tightens as both ends are pulled, the lower spine will align. Through trial and error, actively tuning into the movement of his body, Erik found a specific routine that was right for him:

It's the decompression breathing along with wide founders, and I just go super deep into that work. It takes about five minutes. What I have to do is tire out the support muscles on the side of your spine. Once I can get those muscles tired to where they can no longer clamp down on my spondy, they finally give up after about five minutes of doing a founder. Then I can go into deep decompression breathing, and the muscles can no longer keep everything so tight. And finally it just lets go, and you hear, it's audible, you hear pop, pop, pop, it's amazing.

I've seen and compared Erik's MRIs, from before and after we developed this routine for him. In the latter, the musculature around his spine was around twice as big. That's because he transferred spinal support to the muscles.

Spinal Stenosis: Tony's Story

Tony Blauer is a combat/mixed martial arts instructor who has been doing combat sports—wrestling, martial arts, boxing—for his whole life, and he's been in pain for as long as he can remember. Sparring with students, he was beaten up thirty or forty times a week, so badly that his speech started to slur, and in both his neck and his elbow, a horrific pain settled in for good.

> My threshold for pain is pretty crazy, but there were times the incessant pain would bring me to tears. It was relentless. Now, I'm not suicidal, but there were times when I remember thinking, *I understand why people living with chronic pain kill themselves. This is insane. Do I have to live like this?*

But no amount of medical attention shed light on the root of his pain.

> I went to doctors and they couldn't find anything, so they were like, "We can do exploratory surgery. We can't see what's there, but obviously with the amount of pain you're in, there's something there." They all mean well, but they're guessing. I feel like in many cases, everyone's guessing.

Tony saw myofascial specialists, acupuncturists, chiropractors, but nothing worked. His hamstrings started seizing up, a feeling he likened to a "sudden piranha attack."

> It was debilitating. I couldn't work out. I couldn't get comfortable in bed, which meant I had trouble sleeping. I tried to keep moving. I've got really nice trails near my house, so I would try to go for a walk. I was walking like a hundred-year-old man. Sometimes a hundred yards in, the pain would be so intense I'd need to squat down to release it.

And there would be many times I'd start to cry. I've been an athlete my whole life and I couldn't even walk without pain.

After he had an especially aggressive deep tissue massage, his face started drooping and he had trouble talking, both symptoms of Bell's palsy, which finally sent him in for an MRI.

They said I had severe stenosis. In the same breath, the doctor said, "Here's some medication, and when do you want to schedule a surgery?" No consideration for an alternative, no suggestions—right into surgery. As someone who is scared shitless of an operation on my neck or back, I left more demoralized than ever.

I was like, chronically depressed. It felt like everything was taken away from me.

I was always searching for some magic fix for my ailments, so pretty regularly I searched online for ideas about pain relief. One day I landed on a video of Eric's TEDx talk. When we connected, he took a look at me and said, "I don't think you need surgery, I think you can fix this. I think this'll work, and I think you should try it." And when you're in chronic pain, that's what you wanna hear, but you also want to hear something with a little more certitude. And then he said, "If it works, you'll have to do it for the rest of your life."

One of Tony's underlying issues is called spinal stenosis. Stenosis occurs when the body responds to force by laying down layers of calcium for stability. Those layers of calcium narrow the spaces within the spine, which puts pressure on the nerves that run through the spinal cord. This happens most frequently in either the lower spine or the neck. Unfortunately for Tony, he had it in both areas.

Conventional treatment is painkillers and, more often than not, surgery. In some cases, they actually remove the back of the vertebral column to relieve the pressure. Unless the case is drastic, I am not a fan of this surgery.

Instead, I've found a solution through movement and posture, utilizing both anchoring and decompression. Adjusting the position of the neck by pulling the chin up and back and positioning the weight of the head correctly actively aligns the spine, engaging the abdomen and even the legs. That Chinese finger trap snaps into place, relieving compression, and creating as much space as possible for the nerves to travel in their ideal pathways. It immediately creates improved neural communication.

When I first started working with him, Tony had a tough time. His body was in bad shape, and the exercises hurt him initially, which made him anxious. So we started really slowly. I got him to agree to hold the poses for one minute, just a few times a day. And we gradually increased the routine from there.

It's important to emphasize what we were doing here, as it's common to all of the stories in this book. Tony was learning how to stress his body in a positive way, so it began to actively adapt to healthier movement and posture. With each recurrence of that same stress, the body responds more and more effectively and efficiently. So that the default became, incrementally, healthier and stronger. In our next chapter, we'll explore how this process of active adaptation works in another modality—heat-based therapy—but for now, let's give Tony, slowly but surely healing, the final word:

> I started noticing little changes. The intensity of my bilateral leg pain started lessening. And it inspired me—I mean, nothing breeds success like success itself. So I did it more, a little more, and a little more—I'd do it five, six, sometimes ten times a day. Just little one-minute hits. Microdoses of Foundation Training. I was walking better. The pain was slowly diminishing.
>
> About three and a half months in, I'm out for a walk, and I'm enjoying myself for the first time in a couple years. So I'm swinging my arms and I'm moving along, and all of a sudden I see a sign about twenty-five yards down the road, and I think—I'm getting goose bumps remembering this—I think, *I feel like running. I wonder if I can run to that sign without pain.*
>
> And I ran. And the pain was there, but I remembered Eric saying to me, "Can you work through the pain? Is it a pain that feels like you're damaging something? Or is it just a pain you're afraid of?" And that distinction was very powerful. So I told myself: *Just breathe through it.*
>
> And I ran. And I was screaming while I'm running. Not "in pain" screaming, but screaming for joy! I wasn't running hard or fast, but I was running! I might have been crying. Right after, I called Eric, and I'm like, "Dude, I just fucking ran!"

CHAPTER 3

Hot and Cold

We've talked a lot about the positive aspects of stressing the body and the mind. By pushing our bodies into stressful situations, we learn to positively adapt, so that the next time we are in a similar situation, we act more efficiently. With each exposure, our efficiency increases. As I said before, taking control of stress and using it to activate positive adaptation is the very definition of health. Hot and cold therapies are two specific ways we can do this.

SAUNA

It turns out that sauna bathing has some of the same effects on our bodies as exercise. Exposure to heat rapidly stresses the body, stimulating the sympathetic nervous system. As our minds and bodies work through that stress and acclimate to the heat, we are optimizing our ability to respond more efficiently the next time we enter the sauna (or encounter other stressors as well). So the same three-part process is at play: open-minded curiosity infusing the process of active adaptation, with greater resilience as the result.

From the outside, you might not think it takes a whole lot of curiosity to get into a sauna and sit around. You might not see much active adaptation occurring in that process, either, or increased resilience when a person finally stumbles out. But that process is very real, a fact to which few people could better attest than Evan Halquist and Jessie Salas. As firefighters, they have both used saunas regularly for years. What's more, they have made sauna believers out of thousands of their coworkers, no small feat considering that firefighters are notoriously suspicious of wellness and training "gimmicks." Here is Evan (age thirty-seven, captain, Los Angeles County Fire Department):

> I've got many missions in the fire service. The first was to introduce Foundation Training, which I've done. The second is saunas. Even with such a busy, demanding life, when I get out of the sauna, I feel more clearheaded and calm.
>
> And so I think what that would do for other firefighters' physical and mental health would be a game changer. The last station I was at, I convinced everybody to get a sauna. Ideally, I would love to see one in every fire station in the country.

Firefighters and first responders have some of the most physically demanding and psychologically stressful jobs on the planet. Imagine having to be ready to spring into action at a moment's notice and not knowing what you'll be faced with when you arrive.

The toll it can take on your body and your mental health is extreme. Injuries are par for the course, and depression and anxiety come with the job. First responders and firefighters are chronically sleep-deprived, and on top of that, have to face things that are traumatic and difficult to process, even if they were in the best mental state. Study after study shows that first responders suffer disproportionately from depression, post-traumatic stress disorder (PTSD), and substance abuse. According to one survey, the rate of contemplated and attempted suicide among EMS providers is roughly ten times the national average. Firefighters face greater risk of on-the-job heart attacks and are significantly more likely to die of cancer than the general population.

Jessie, who was a firefighter in Orlando for seventeen years before he became chief Foundation trainer, remembers how that pressure felt, day to day, and how a sauna helped release that:

When you've left a really stressful shift or you've dealt with some really traumatic stuff, it's pent up—and, you know, guys will deny it, guys won't talk about it, and even I never fully understood how much the calls affected me until I left the fire career. After a shift, most guys are in this high-wired state. They have an immune system that's beaten down, a body that's stuck in a high-sympathetic state all the time, and they don't even realize it. Then they get in traffic and can't handle it when someone pulls out in front of them. Or they go home and get in a fight with their wife. It's very common—road rage, marital issues, because they have no fuse anymore, you know? But when you get in a sauna, you're essentially elevating the heart rate, you're sweating everything out, and then going home and going to bed.

Evan, who has tracked the long-term difference that saunas have made for his coworkers, observes: "At Fire Station 131, the guys reported lower stress levels, an increase in the ability to think clearly in stressful situations, an increase in their cardiorespiratory condition, and fewer overall illnesses, like colds and the flu." Those are concrete and dramatic changes.

If even anecdotally, saunas can help maintain the physical and mental well-being for firefighters, who are under constant, extreme stress, just imagine how effectively they could help us adapt to the more routine stressors of daily life!

We'll talk about the medical benefits of this practice shortly, but first let's look at its long and incredible history. Sauna is not some recent trend; we've been doing it forever.

SWEATING THROUGH HISTORY

Back in 2000 BC, in Northern Europe, the first saunas were simple man-made caves, draped with animal skins and heated by a fire underneath a pile of rocks. The rocks absorbed and maintained the heat, and when water was poured on them, it created purifying steam. Those early saunas were for much more than relaxing, too; they were the place where food was prepared and illness was treated, where families found shelter and warmth for entire winters. Similarly, sweat lodges still play a crucial part in North American Native American culture, the center of ceremonies used to cleanse and purify the mind, body, spirit, and emotions. Wherever and whenever it unfolded, the history of the sauna is the history of people just trying to feel better, physically, emotionally, and spiritually.

While the tradition has held strong in places like Finland and

Russia, the Enlightenment—which called for reason and logic over mysticism and spirituality—led to a massive decline in sauna use. But by the mid-twentieth century, this ancient practice of using heat for purification, cleansing, and healing had made a comeback, with saunas found in health clubs and spas. Still, despite sauna's ancient origins, science has been slow to catch on, and there have not been nearly enough studies investigating the health benefits of the practice. Those that have been conducted, however, show extremely promising results.

SAUNAS AND HEALTH

Given the history, it's no surprise that the longest-running study about the medical benefits of sauna bathing, as it's called, comes from eastern Finland. The Kuopio Ischaemic Heart Disease Risk Factor (KIHD) Study has tracked more than 2,300 middle-aged men, starting in the 1980s, for over twenty years. In the 1990s, women of a similar age were recruited as well. Participants have been reexamined four, eleven, and twenty years after their baseline vitals were established, and the study is still ongoing. The results have been extraordinary and have spurred almost 500 international, peer-reviewed articles.

So what exactly was being examined? Pretty much everything: individual behaviors, lifestyle, psychological profiles, early life histories, cognitive functioning, ECG measurements, exercise tests, atherosclerosis (buildup of cholesterol plaque on artery walls), and lots of other health markers, both physical and mental. One of the major takeaways is that men who used the sauna two to three times a week were 27 percent less likely to die from cardiovascular-related causes than men who didn't use the sauna. Even more extraordinary, the more you sauna bathe, the more it helps. Men who used the sauna twice as often (four to seven times a week) experienced roughly twice the benefits. They were 50 percent less likely to die from cardiovascular-related diseases. In fact, frequent sauna users were found to be 40 percent less likely to die *from all cases of premature death*. That statistic held true even when age, activity level, and other lifestyle factors were considered.

If that's not compelling enough, sauna bathing has also been shown to have significant health effects beyond the cardiovascular system. Men who used the sauna four to seven times a week had a 66 percent lower risk of developing dementia and a 65 percent lower risk of developing Alzheimer's disease, compared to men who used the sauna only once a week. And the mental health benefits are just as profound. Sauna bathing four to seven times a week resulted in a 77 percent less chance of developing psychotic disorders, regardless of dietary habits, socioeconomic status, or level of physical activity.

The sauna sessions in the study were found to be most effective when they lasted around twenty minutes, at a temperature of at least 174° F. In fact, the study concluded that a longer stay in the sauna (as opposed to a shorter stay of between eleven and nineteen minutes) positively affected the cardiovascular benefits.

The study and its follow-ups show conclusively that sauna bathing improves our cardiovascular health, prevents cardiovascular disease and congestive heart failure, lowers hypertension, and decreases cellular inflammation, which plays a vital role in many chronic diseases, including cancer and diabetes. Sauna baths have also been shown to boost our natural painkilling process (particularly when it comes to arthritis and headaches) and to help us recover from the flu. In terms of our mental health, sauna bathing slows cognitive decline, alleviates depression, increases focus and attention span, and improves exercise performance. These are some pretty remarkable results.

TAKE THE HEAT: THE SCIENCE OF STRESS IN SAUNA

Let's get into why sitting in a hot box might have so many positive benefits. What happens inside us with exposure to all that heat?

The cardiovascular response is immediate. In this system, three crucial things occur: our cardiac output (the amount of work the heart performs due to our need for oxygen) increases by 60 to 70 percent; our heart rate increases; and while the amount of blood pumped remains the same, anywhere from 50 to 70 percent of our blood flow is redistributed from the core to the skin, to help with sweating.

Over time, sauna bathing acclimates the body to heat and optimizes our future exposure. This is due to something called hormesis, "a compensatory defense response following exposure to a mild stressor that is disproportionate to the magnitude of the stressor." In layman's terms, that just means little effort, great reward. Hormesis initiates a host of mechanisms that repair cell damage and offer protection from later exposures to even more harmful sources of stress. Not surprisingly, this is the same physiological response that occurs during mild to moderate exercise.

Hormesis is facilitated by the increased activation of heat shock proteins, which are present in all cells. They play a vital role in many processes, including immune function and cell regulation. Damaged proteins, which can clump together, are implicated in cardiovascular disease, Alzheimer's disease, and Parkinson's disease. During what's called the heat shock response, heat proteins become more active, preventing this clumping and repairing proteins that have been damaged. Simply put, elevating the temperature of our body initiates a chain of extremely beneficial reactions that improve our health.

Increasing the heat in our body is very metabolically intense and muscularly dependent. The elevated blood flow and decreased blood viscosity loosens up our muscles, providing them with hydration. The same thing occurs in our spinal discs: increased blood flow and hydration, but without the increased force on the spine that can occur during exercise. A lot of the pain relief we see from heat is just what happens when the blood starts pumping faster with enough hydration. Your body repurposes some of the water in the interstitial areas, between cells, pulling it into the tissue that needs it.

The one thing that occurs immediately when you enter a sauna, as soon as your heart rate increases by 20 percent or so, is that you just feel different. You're clearer, less depressed, less anxious, more focused. Right away, there is this shift in the internal concentration of your body, as fluid gets pulled into muscles and you start to sweat. You feel your glands open up, and there's a legitimate neurological shift in all of your bodily functions. You very quickly become calm.

But as the heat increases, your body ramps right back up, stimulating the fight-or-flight response of your parasympathetic nervous system. You start to feel a little anxious and sweat profusely. You are inducing a stress response, and your body is learning how to efficiently adapt to it. The longer your body can stay there, the longer it can register what's happening and improve upon that registry. That's thanks, in no small part, to the endogenous cannabinoid system (which we'll discuss in the next chapter), the system that modulates the body's response to stress and teaches it to adapt to larger physical stresses.

SWEAT IT OUT: SAUNA AND DETOX

The health and wellness industry is big on the concept of detox. But detoxification is more complicated than commonly believed, and no special tea is going to achieve it for us, no matter how it is marketed. The liver is in charge of detoxifying our blood, and if it's healthy, it does a great job. But along with the liver, our lymphatic system is also a major detoxification pathway for the body, removing toxins from its tissues.

Here's what Evan has to say:

I do training burns at the fire academy, where we sit inside a room that's filled with smoke for hours. I walk out of there smelling like smoke; it's just seeping off my skin. I'll have brain fog from all the carbon monoxide I inhale. When I work out, I'll smell it in my sweat. It's the same when I fight a structure or brush fire. But when I use the sauna, it lessens that. So in my own experience, it helps tremendously.

And here's Jessie:

You're walking around fire trucks all day, and the body's absorbing the diesel and benzene. And they're finding that even the materials used as fire retardants in the firefighting gear causes cancer. When you go into a fire, wearing all that gear, your body's just absorbing everything. Saunas really allow the body to detox and sweat out the crap. We take hot showers after a fire, and your pores open up and you smell the smoke. Even when you're wearing air masks, the next day we'd be picking black soot boogers out of our noses.

While most of us don't deal with the chemical exposure that firefighters do, we are all still bombarded with environmental and food toxins, as well as chemicals in our personal care products. Sweating helps cleanse the body of certain toxins (including heavy metals; BPA, which is found in plastic; and PCBs, which although now illegal, are still found in the environment) that accumulate in the muscle, adipose tissue, and organ tissue. Sauna bathing triggers and activates the body's natural detoxification pathways—sweating and lymphatic drainage. In particular, the lymphatic system (a network of tissues, vessels, and organs that move a watery fluid called lymph back into our circulatory system) has enormous detoxifying properties. It collects excess fluid that drains from cells and tissues throughout the body and returns it to the bloodstream, absorbs fats from the digestive tract, and transports and removes waste products and abnormal cells. Between the cardiovascular, mental health, and detox benefits, the stress response that sauna bathing induces affects almost all of our bodily systems.

TECHNIQUES OF SAUNA

Saunas were traditionally heated with wood, and sometimes still are, particularly in northern Finland. It's the most economical way to enjoy the benefits of a sauna (more on that later), and there is something profoundly satisfying about building a fire for this purpose. Certainly more convenient are electric versions, which warm the air to between 158°F and 220°F. The heat of the air then transfers to the body, working from the outside in to eventually raise your core temperature. Infrared heaters, which operate at lower temperatures, work the opposite way: using thermal radiation to heat the body directly, from the inside out. This technology relies on many sources of infrared light, so that numerous rays collectively heat the body and the heat can penetrate more deeply than traditional saunas.

If possible, I ask my patients to sauna bathe three or four times a week as part of their therapy. Getting in a sauna, detoxing, and perspiring—that in and of itself gives people a tremendous amount of relief, mentally and physically.

A few things to note. Sauna is not recommended if you're pregnant. If you are on pain medications that stimulate the opioid system, sauna is not recommended, either. Those drugs make you feel less, and while you therefore are able to tolerate more heat, that is not necessarily what your body needs. If you are prescribed multiple medications, their interaction—with each other and with the environment of the sauna—can be unpredictable. So do your research, talk to your doctor, and try to work with him or her to minimize your medications.

Once you're in the sauna, you must hydrate during the process. I usually suggest drinking at least an additional liter of water before you get in.

You will need to build up your endurance, in terms of heat and duration. The first twelve times you use the sauna, it should be for less than twenty minutes, and you should keep the temperature under 190°F. Let yourself get used to it. 175°F to 185°F for twenty minutes is a legitimate goal. The idea is to start slowly and not push yourself to extremes.

From there, you just ramp up slowly, at your own pace. Keep in mind that the last ten minutes should really challenge you, and you are going to contend with some panicky thoughts: *Whew, I don't feel good. I think I should go. I think I gotta get out!* Every single person who stays in a sauna long enough goes through this. Your eyes close a lot. When this happens, even an extra thirty seconds of calm breathing will help you push through and make the next time you approach sauna therapy more controllable, more manageable. Again, that's the work of the endogenous cannabinoid system, which regulates pulse, respiration, and temperature.

Throughout the sauna bath process, the concept of curiosity applies. Listen and tune in to your body. That includes generalized somatosensation—taking stock of your heart rate, your breathing rate, and your posture. If you are within even 10 percent of your max heart rate, it's time to get out. No questions asked.

Think of the sauna not as a sprint, but an uphill hike with no downhill portion. Don't try to "come down" in the sauna. Once you're at the peak, you exit.

FROM SAUNA TO LIFE

The skill of sauna happens in those first twelve to twenty times—recognizing how your body responds to heat and understanding that your first sensations of anxiety do not mean you have to get out. That takes real mental training. You're learning about your stress response and your anxiety by confronting and overcoming it.

This involves working, intelligently, against instinct. We are designed for self-preservation, so when it comes to feelings of pain and stress, we can be overly cautious. But when we push ever so slightly past those boundaries of perceived self-preservation, in a smart and healthy way, that's when we experience pleasure and reward.

The better you become at that specific decision to push, the better you get at decision-making in general. You're testing your will, just like you would exercise a muscle, increasing your ability to maintain your composure in moments of frustration, teaching yourself to make a positive decision in the face of adversity. We use that muscle of resolve and perseverance in all kinds of decisions, when it comes to our health and life more generally. It's a discipline, and if you stay with it, pain relief seems easier, exercise seems easier, and emotional issues seem easier, too.

This process, of course, is the same one involved in the strength, movement, posture, and breathing work we discussed. These modalities are all centered around microdosing stress in order to alleviate future stress. The better you get at the skill of biomechanics, at learning how to properly align yourself and move efficiently, the better you become at absorbing your body's weight in real time. That manifests itself in everything you do: standing, sitting, walking, even sleeping. Likewise, when you heat up your body, you are expending calories trying to cool off, and you're learning to get better at not being stressed during the process. You are also teaching your mind how to better handle that stress (and similar stresses) in the future.

Indeed, research suggests that this process of purposeful stressing can lead to more global resilience—the ability to handle different kinds of stresses—by improving our cognitive reserve, the brain's ability to improvise and problem-solve. A recent study with mice, published in *Translational Psychiatry*, suggests that "stress inocula-tion training may enhance cognitive reserve, which in turn improves coping across multiple stress contexts."

In fact, both sauna therapy and Foundation Training consume energy that might otherwise be expended by less healthy bodily functions, namely mental rumination. That is because mental rumi-nation is extraordinarily taxing on the body. As an extreme example, Robert Sapolsky, who teaches biology and neurology at Stanford and studies stress in primates, says professional chess players can burn up to 6,000 calories a day during a tournament, three times the normal rate, due to the elevated breathing and blood rates and mus-cle contractions that go along with competition. In fact, the 1984 World Chess Championship was called off after five months and forty-eight games because defending champion Anatoly Karpov had lost twenty-two pounds. Of course, ordinary mental rumination doesn't come with such extreme physiological changes, but it does take its toll, especially cumulatively over the course of a day.

With heat, we're taking stress and using that energy and pushing it out—instead of mental rumination, instead of physical motion—through sweat. In Foundation Training, we actively contract mus-cles to support body weight in motion and at rest. These are both intense metabolic expenditures, which we incur as we develop a very useful skill: the skill of positive adaptation.

TAKE THE (COLD) PLUNGE

You've probably seen pictures of people running from an outdoor sauna and rolling in the snow or hurling themselves into an icy stream. Or you've seen movies where professional athletes are submerged in an ice bath after a particularly rough match. So let's move from hot to cold and examine the benefits of cold therapy.

In some ways, using ice for injuries and injury prevention is more accepted than heat therapy, but I don't think it's nearly as important. Still, there is a place for it in a healthy lifestyle, and many people do swear by it, particularly to reduce inflammation.

For me, the perfect level of cold therapy is winter surfing in Santa Barbara. The water is a shock, but it's not actually freezing—about 52°F to 55°F. You can go in without a wet suit if you're brave, and you're not going to get hypothermia during a quick surf session even if you're afraid you might. It's the same as staying in the sauna for those final ten minutes: you think you can't make it, but you can.

There's been a shift in the scientific view of cold and ice therapy over the last ten years. Most often, people are using this treatment because of injuries and/or pain, both of which either cause or are a result of increased inflammation. When tissue is submerged in the cold, it constricts, which might seem to address the issue. But the blood that is being pushed out is eventually going to come rushing back in, bringing with it a storm of inflammatory chemicals. So the long-term effect of ice is not necessarily all that beneficial. The old formula of RICE (rest, ice, compression, and elevation) that used to be taught in first aid courses is now simply rest, compress, and elevate.

But even if cold therapy is no longer prescribed as it once was, it's still beneficial in short windows for the nervous system and for our mental health. In just five or six minutes, an ice bath can reset you, and the lasting effects are wonderful. Here's how Evan starts his day before driving into the fire station.

The first thing I do when I get up in the morning is roll out of bed and jump in an ice bath for a few minutes. It might seem like the worst way to start your day, but the reason why it's so great is that no matter what happens, the rest of the day is easier when compared to that. I absolutely love it. It's definitely a mental challenge, but you check that box first thing in the morning, and you're good to go.

Jackson Fortunato, a martial arts master, needed a little more convincing. While at a five-day jiujitsu retreat, he was informed that they would be taking ice baths, but thought it was a joke before he saw the truck full of ice.

I freaked out because I never liked the cold. I'm from Brazil! I like sunshine! I went into the ice bath and nearly died after two minutes. But as I was gasping, the instructor walked by me and said, "Jackson! Just breathe and relax." And that is what I've been telling my jiujitsu students for my whole career. When they freak out in the fight, I say, "Hey, chill out! Take your time; save energy to defeat the bigger guy." When he said that, I did relax, and I stayed there for the remainder of the time. That's exactly what I do in jiujitsu—survive in chaos. When you go inside the ice, it's immediately chaos, and you have to master that in your head, and it's going to be good for you.

What Jackson is describing is active adaptation: pushing his body just a little bit past his comfort zone, stressing it so that it learns how to respond efficiently.

When I came back home, I started to do ice baths all the time. I'd invite all my students to my house, and ice bath was my new thing. I had suffered from tendinitis in my elbows for more than ten years. I had tried all kinds of treatments—cortisone, platelet injections, you name it. After I started doing ice baths, I noticed that my tendinitis was healing. And now the pain and inflammation are just gone. I like being exposed to the cold now, and I feel like I wasted years avoiding it. It's not an enemy anymore. So the big thing was reeducating me about something that I was always so negative about.

For some devotees of sauna, there is a strong appeal in moving from that extreme hot to extreme cold. But you do need to be careful. If you move back and forth more than three times, you're burning out your nervous system, expending all your adrenaline intensely. Even if you think you've cooled down after a cold shower, your core is still heated, and you need a few hours to completely cool down before heating back up again. Getting thrown such mixed signals, your brain and central nervous system get stuck between cooling off and heating up. Then, because you've drained all your adrenaline, you'll spend the next forty-eight hours exhausted and utterly depleted. That's more like recovery from trauma than recovery from training.

EVEN IF YOU'RE A MOUTH-BREATHER

One of the main ways to reap the benefits of staying in slightly uncomfortable situations, hot or cold, is to focus on your breath. I've gone on at length about decompression breathing in the previous chapter, and I truly think this is one of the most important things I have to offer. Learning to breathe in a way that expands your torso, fills your lungs to capacity, and widens the thoracic cage will have a profound impact on your overall health and mood.

Practicing this technique in the sauna increases the intensity a bit, along with the results. When our bodies are hot, vasodilation occurs: the diameter of our pulmonary veins and arteries increases, and with every breath we take, we increase our blood oxygenation; our increased heart rate pumps that oxygen around more quickly. Everyone knows from science class that breathing replaces the carbon dioxide in your lungs with fresh oxygen, which enters the bloodstream and is circulated throughout the body. The more efficient we are at this, the better and deeper we breathe, the cleaner that exchange is.

There's also some fascinating new science that underscores the need not just for healthy breathing, but for healthy lungs. Recent studies have found that platelets, once thought to originate only in bone marrow, are also generated in the lungs. There are 150 to 450 billion platelets in every liter of blood, and their lifespan is only eight to ten days. Every day, we turn over 100 billion platelets to maintain the proper concentrate. Those platelets play a crucial role in wound healing and immunity. It only makes sense that better breathing means better lung capacity, which means more effective and efficient platelet production.

THE WIM HOF METHOD

I ask my patients to get as much oxygen in their system when they first enter the sauna as they can, and to do this, I recommend the

Wim Hof breathing method: big, deep, fast breaths that really purge the carbon dioxide from your lungs and replace it with fresh oxygen.

The method is named after its very colorful inventor: Wim Hof, a well-weathered Dutchman in his sixties who has run a half-marathon barefoot and shirtless, *above the Arctic Circle*. He climbed Mount Kilimanjaro wearing only shorts and shoes. He remained submerged in an ice bath for 112 minutes. It won't come as a surprise that his nickname is the Iceman. But the Iceman also tackled the heat, running a half-marathon (with no training) through the Namib Desert without drinking any water.

He attributes these record-breaking feats to his particular method of breathing. Remember when Jackson was having a panic attack in the ice bath at his jiujitsu retreat? The instructor told him to practice Wim Hof breathing, and it allowed him to stay the course.

The method is actually quite simple. Just like decompression breathing, you can do it anywhere, not just when you are sauna bathing or challenging your body by taking a dip in a freezing lake. Take thirty quick, deep breaths, inhaling through your nose and exhaling through your mouth. They should feel quite rapid. Then take as deep a breath as you can, and then exhale. Hold until you need to breathe in. Inhale again, as deeply as you can, and hold for ten seconds. That's it. Wim Hof recommends repeating this pattern three to five times.

Nobody explains or teaches it as well as he does, so I encourage you to check out his work. It's an extremely energizing practice, and great to do in the morning or before a workout. I find that practicing this method for the first few minutes I'm in a sauna (or even before I get in) intensifies the experience. Do not attempt to engage this method after you've been in the sauna for even five minutes. It will heat you up too fast.

Why does it work? Breathing is part of our autonomic nervous system; like our heartbeat and digestion, it happens unconsciously. Many people pay no attention to their breath at all and consequently suffer from shallow breathing.

But we can also *consciously* engage with our breath, taking control. The Wim Hof Method (like many controlled hyperventilation methods) forces us to be aware of our breathing and offers an intriguing link between our subconscious mind and our physiology. If we control our breathing, what other processes or internal states could we control? Breathing with awareness is at the fulcrum of the mind-body connection, and exploring that, Wim Hof believes, leads to many health benefits.

When scientists did an MRI on his brain, they found that he was able to consciously induce a stress response and trigger a natural painkiller function that helps him overcome the effects of the cold. Not only could he stand staying in the cold, but he actually felt euphoric.

By consciously engaging our mind-body connection, we can push through the primal fear that wants us to run from discomfort. The more we do it, the better we adapt to it, and the easier it is the next time. And like sauna bathing, we take this practice into our daily lives, when other stressors threaten to derail us.

THE BUTEYKO METHOD

There is a point of diminishing health returns in the sauna, however, a threshold when the heart is beating too fast and you can't get enough oxygen with every breath to match every pump. At that point, you have to slow down. You've oxygenated your blood and it's time to relax. Again, it is all about maintaining awareness of your heart rate and breath and knowing when to push yourself and when to back off. When your heart rate has increased to the point where you feel like you're jogging, it's time to calm down, and we switch to something called the Buteyko breathing technique.

The Buteyko breathing technique is named for Konstantin Pavlovich Buteyko, a Soviet doctor who developed it in the 1950s. It focuses on breathing through the nose only, as the nasal passages protect the airways by humidifying, warming, and cleaning the air before it enters the lungs. The breaths employed here are basically the opposite of Wim Hof: barely perceptible and relaxing rather than energizing. You can bring more awareness to the process by pinching one nostril, inhaling, then switching nostrils and exhaling out the other. I find it brings great awareness to the process and really works to quiet the mind just when you are starting to feel a little anxiety about the heat. At this point, our sympathetic nervous system has kicked into gear, and we have to push through to reap the benefits of the stress we are putting our body under.

Here's trainer Pat Helma on his own experience with breathing, sauna, cold, and active adaptation, all together:

I do decompression breathing and some breath work while I'm in the sauna. That last five minutes becomes a real bitch, because I want to get out. When I'm done, I'll just step outside on the porch, where it's usually about 20 degrees in the winter, and I'll just sit out there for a couple of minutes and cool down. I like the idea of contrast and trying to get the body used to changes. We want to make our body as adaptable as we can. So if we get into a difficult situation, our body is like, "Yeah, I got that." You've got to kind of push yourself in things. It helps the body become more resilient.

If this sounds too intense or complicated, don't let that scare you away from sauna bathing. Remember Josh Holland, who uses Foundation techniques to help with his scoliosis? He mostly just chills out in the sauna.

I will admit, I'm not as deep into the breath work as I might be. It's like, bro, I want to just relax in here. I want my sauna session to be meditative and relaxing, but I usually start that out with some sort of breath work or decompression breathing to set that up.

DO IT ON THE CHEAP

If you're interested in incorporating saunas or cold therapy into your life, don't get put off by the price. Beautiful saunas (indoors and out) are fantastic, but they are expensive. They're a good investment and last a lifetime, but there are much cheaper alternatives. There are great little personal saunas available for around a hundred dollars, and tent saunas that require building a fire for between $500 and $1,200. Patti Sheaff doesn't even have room for those, and instead uses infrared mats and blankets to raise her body temperature. However you do it, the benefits of adding heat to your wellness routine are worth it.

Likewise, there is no need to pay hundreds of dollars to sit in a cryotherapy chamber to chill your body. Evan made his ice bath out of a large chest freezer, simply by sealing the inner edges and joints with caulking so it doesn't leak. Even a bracingly cold shower will do the trick if you stay in it long enough.

Incorporating these elements into your life, particularly saunas, is going to have immeasurable benefits. Those old guys in Finland? They are still being studied. Think of the things we are going to learn as they head toward their senior years, healthy and happy. In the meantime, sauna fans like Jessie Salas can teach us plenty. Compared to the Fins, Jessie may be a newbie, but his insights are invaluable:

The sauna takes your brain to a point of discomfort where we all want to get out, right? And so I look at it as, yeah, you're sweating, you're detoxing, you're feeding something very important—but you're also going to take your brain to this moment of discomfort. The underlying fact is that when you challenge the brain, you challenge the body to go to that point of discomfort, and you come out of there, it changes the way the brain is and how you meet the day. You're elevating the heart rate, you're sweating everything out, you're feeding some very important systems of the body. There's value in that and the mental reset that comes from it—and it doesn't take a large amount of effort.

CHAPTER 4

Nourishing the Endocannabinoid System

Let's zero in on something Jessie Salas just said at the end of the last chapter: "[W]hen you challenge the brain, you challenge the body to go to that point of discomfort, and you come out of there, it changes the way the brain is and how you meet the day." And in chapter 2, remember what Tony Blauer said about his work with Foundation Training poses and breathing exercises, purposefully taking his body into the experience of momentary pain to alleviate chronic pain: "I started noticing little changes . . . And it inspired me . . . So I did it more, a little more, and a little more . . . Just little one-minute hits."

Both experiences underscore a process that is thematically central to this book: inquisitive engagement with sensation (curiosity) fuels active adaptation (changing through intentionally induced stress), which increases resilience (the mind and body's improved ability to meet future stress). As we'll see in this chapter, there is an actual system in our bodies that fuels this process, enabling us to become stronger and more efficient through stress. In order to strengthen and optimize that process, we need to support, stimulate, and nourish the underlying system in a vigorous and strategic way.

We've talked a lot about complacent versus active adaptation, which is a choice we make for ourselves. We either passively allow our bodies to adopt poor movement patterns or we teach ourselves to change in a positive, healthy direction. Awareness is the first step. But once we activate those positive adaptations, how exactly do they work?

Think about those extra ten seconds you have challenged yourself to add on during some of the Foundation Training poses, or the first time you drove a car, when you're battling a little bit of anxiety to keep going. As they happen, those moments are transcribed and registered in the body, so that the next time they occur, your body is more prepared to meet the challenge.

The system that helps to mitigate unnecessary energy and stress expenditures is called the endogenous cannabinoid system (ECS). Endogenous means internal. Cannabinoids refer to chemicals that bind to specific receptors in our bodies and brains in a similar manner to chemicals found in the cannabis plant. We'll talk about how the ECS got its name shortly.

It is an ancient system, having evolved in animals over 500 million years ago. But we didn't know it existed until 1992. Since then, we have been quickly learning more about its roles in our body. Besides how it helps us to adapt to stress, our ECS regulates and makes more efficient a host of essential bodily functions: pain perception, immune function, motor control, fertility, memory, sleep, hunger, pleasure, mood, temperature, metabolism, and cardiovascular activity, just to list a few. On an overall level, the ECS helps us to maintain homeostasis, which is balance or equilibrium between interdependent bodily processes and systems—cardiovascular, lymphatic, neurological, and reproductive.

Now let's look back at how this system got its name.

A HIDDEN SYSTEM, DISCOVERED

Our understanding of this "hidden system" has a long and fascinating history, beginning thousands of years ago, when ancient cultures started ingesting the cannabis plant for recreational and medicinal uses. We don't know precisely when this started, but in 2019, archaeologists found definitive proof of the earliest consumption yet known: 2,500-year-old traces of burned cannabis at a mountaintop cemetery in western China, evidence suggesting that an early society of Zoroastrians were using the plant in a religious ritual. As the plant spread, first via trade along the Silk Road, its mind-altering and medicinal properties were shared by more and more cultures across Asia, the Middle East, and beyond.

Starting in the late nineteenth century, scientists began to investigate the chemistry of this wondrous plant more systematically. In 1964, a team of Israeli scientists led by Dr. Raphael Mechoulam isolated two compounds inside cannabis which Mechoulam called cannabinoids—tetrahydrocannabinol (THC) and cannabidiol (CBD).

Mechoulam's discovery launched decades of study into how, at a molecular level, THC worked in the human brain. In 1988, a team at the St. Louis University Medical School discovered specialized receptor sites in rats' brains that are activated by THC. One such receptor, named CB1, was subsequently found to be extremely abundant in all mammalian brains, greater in number than any other similarly structured cell-surface receptors. The questions and implications of this revelation were huge. Why do we have the built-in ability to respond to cannabinoids from outside the body? Scientists realized that we must have something like THC inside our own bodies that triggers CB1 receptors, too. We must have our own naturally produced cannabinoids.

Sure enough, in 1992, that's just what Mechoulam and others discovered: a cannabinoid neurotransmitter produced by the body that binds with CB1 like THC does. They named it anandamide, after the Sanskrit word *ananda*, which means joy or bliss. When anandamide, just like THC, triggers CB1, it sparks a lot more than just changes in mood. The cannabinoids effect changes in cells that regulate appetite, perception of pain, and fertility; they enable the creation of new brain cells.

A year later came the discovery of another cannabinoid receptor, CB2, that regulates the body's immune system and inflammation, among other things. In subsequent years, more receptors were discovered, not just present in the brain and nerves, as initially thought, but in tissue throughout our bodies, from our skin and bone to our blood vessels and immune cells to our kidneys, gastrointestinal tract, and heart. Pain, mood, stress, sleep, metabolism, and immune and reproductive function . . . Discovery by discovery, the picture began to emerge of an entire cannabinoid system—working everywhere in the body and controlling all of its vital systems and processes.

So the name *cannabinoid* came from the plant, which was studied first, and then was given to the bodily system, which was understood later—not unlike how the term *opiate receptors* came from opium. So, whether or not we have ever consumed cannabinoids or opiates, these compounds are in our bodies, naturally produced. And they always have been there; we are born with our endocannabinoid system intact and fully functioning. That means, with proper guidance and knowledge, it is something we can tap into. Humans aren't the only ones who have this system, either: it turns out endocannabinoids are produced by all vertebrates and some invertebrates, too.

THE ECS, ADAPTATION, AND HOMEOSTASIS

Taken broadly, the ECS helps regulate homeostasis: the stability of our internal environment. It coordinates how our nervous system, immune system, hormonal system, and organs respond to external and internal stress. It does that by registering and recording the stressful stimulus after it occurs, and then making our response to future exposures to that stimulus more efficient and effective. If an outside force, such as pain, throws our body off-balance, the ECS kicks in to help restore the equilibrium. If we are introducing positive stress, like challenging Foundation poses, each time the ECS returns us to homeostasis, we are in a slightly improved position. Our body has learned to meet the stress head-on, so that next time we can handle just a little bit more. Simply put, stimulation of the ECS helps us positively adapt.

Think about exercise. Adaptation comes because you're stressing your body to a point where it needs to change—produce a new response to pain, a new way to move or breathe—in order to complete the workout. That change occurs molecularly, at a chemical level. Every time you push yourself just a little bit further, your body rewards you by creating anandamide, a chemical that pushes the button of pleasure. Your body begins to expect that pleasure the next time you push it toward stress. In addition, with experience, you find that your pain and fear diminish as well. The more you encounter that same stress, the easier it gets. That's because you've repeated those minor stresses a little more frequently, so that your body is responding more efficiently. Remember Tony Blauer, who could hold some of the Foundation poses for only a brief time. Even that short routine, practiced steadily over time, was enough to stress his body into making positive changes. That is your endogenous cannabinoid system, doing its job: making our everyday adaptations more and more efficient.

I'd like to underscore the personal agency involved in this process. All too often, homeostasis is thought of as this perfect ecosystem that the body just achieves and maintains on its own, internally, regardless of what we do or don't do. It's true that our bodies have many involuntary processes. But we also have the ability to improve those processes. So I describe homeostasis as an active, resilient recentering of the body's interdependent systems, with you in charge: the more you practice throwing yourself off-balance, the better you get at returning to balance. Off-balance to on-balance—it's that simple.

The better you get at this, the hardier you become, regardless of the physical or mental stress coming at you. The ECS helps your body learn how to react productively. And that "reward" feeling of homeostasis is what keeps us coming back for more; it's how we shift from complacent adaptation to active adaptation. When Tony spotted that sign and decided to run for it, he purposefully threw himself way off-balance, and when he started, he screamed in agony because he anticipated feeling weak and being in pain. The journey seemed impossible. But once he made it to the sign, he cried tears of joy. The euphoria of that accomplishment—his reward—kept him coming back to run farther and farther the next time. By pushing through, he conditioned his body to be stronger so that the next time it was a little easier to go a bit farther, and the next time it was easier still. Finally he got to the point where he could move with more agility and less pain.

THE SCIENCE BEHIND THE SYSTEM

Now that you've been introduced to the ECS, I want to explain how it relates to your ability to self-heal. For that we need to go a little deeper into science.

The ECS consists of three interrelated parts. The first components are the cannabinoid receptors, found in every tissue type in the body. In the brain, CB1 receptors are found in the cortex, basal ganglia, hippocampus, cerebellum, thalamus, and amygdala. In the spinal cord, receptors are found within the dorsal horn, the column of gray matter at the posterior of the spine. The dorsal horn is where somatosensory input travels; it contains the neurons that receive and transmit *every sensation* our body processes, from head to the toes. CB1 receptors (and CB2 receptors to a lesser degree) are in the lungs and bronchial tissue, and both types are found in the heart and cardiovascular tissues. CB2 receptors are everywhere, from the immune system to the reproductive system, from the liver and kidney to blood cells and bones and gut to the surface of the skin.

The second component of the ECS are the endocannabinoids

themselves, the primary variations being anandamide and 2-arachi-donoylglycerol, or 2-AG. Endocannabinoids are produced naturally, in various parts of the body and brain, in response to all kinds of environmental stimuli like stress, pain, and hunger. They bind with the cannabinoid receptors, like a key in a lock, sparking a further chemical response in the central nervous system, which addresses that original stimulus-reducing stress, alleviating pain, stimulating appetite, working to return the body to homeostasis.

The third component is the various enzymes that break the cannabinoids down after they've done their job, the cleanup crew. The entire process is precise and targeted, impacting only the specific bodily processes that are out of balance.

To really understand how the ECS is unique among bodily systems, let's look more closely at just how endocannabinoids work. Most of our body's neurotransmitters travel from one neuron through a synapse to another neuron, then attach to a receptor in that "receiver" postsynaptic neuron, which reacts and passes the message forward to the next neuron. But not endocannabinoids. They are rebellious, moving in the opposite direction, from post-synaptic neuron across the synapse to the presynaptic neuron, where they bind to receptors. So the signal is backward—transmitted from the periphery toward the central nervous system and brain. Reverse engineering at its best.

There's a really good reason for this. When cannabinoids bind to those presynaptic receptors, they impact how that neuron later reacts. In moments of intense pain, our neurons first bombard the brain with pain signals. But cannabinoids, when they attach to those neurons, keep them occupied or "full," lessening how many pain signals they can transmit to the brain. Fewer pain signals means less pain. Since cannabinoids act on presynaptic cells, they can control what happens next when these cells are activated. Think of cannabinoids as kind of a dimmer switch for the release of neurotransmitters.

THE ECS: SYSTEM BY SYSTEM

I've mentioned the range of bodily functions that the ECS helps to regulate; now let's take a closer look. In all of these systems, the ECS is constantly at work keeping bodily functions in balance, activating with targeted responses that are just enough to get the job done.

In our immune system, the ECS plays a huge role in controlling inflammation, which is our body's natural way of protecting itself in response to physical damage or infection. In a healthy immune response, fluid and immune cells flood into an affected area and get rid of damaged tissue and germs, stopping once the issue is resolved. It's the ECS that strictly governs that response, how long it lasts and how widespread it is. Problems can arise when the immune system is overactivated, when those immune cells don't stop flooding in, creating chronic inflammation and any number of autoimmune diseases. By regulating this entire process, the ECS keeps everything in check.

Within the central nervous system, the ECS works to limit or inhibit other neurotransmitters, an excess of which can cause any number of disorders and imbalances. The ECS balances the transmission of glutamate, responsible for stimulating the system, with the transmission of GABA (a neurotransmitter that sends chemical messages through the brain and the nervous system and is involved in regulating communication between brain cells), which is responsible for calming the system down. When this balance is off, we're prone to be foggy and muddled (too much GABA), or anxious, scattered, antisocial, or combative (too much glutamate). In addition, an extreme excess of glutamate can lead to Parkinson's, schizophrenia, migraines, restless legs syndrome, multiple sclerosis, or epilepsy. Also in the nervous system, the ECS is a key player in creating new neurons, which are essential for neural plasticity, the ability of the nervous system to change, adapt, and reorganize.

In the digestive system, the ECS helps keep hunger in check, stimulating our appetite only when the body needs nutrients. It also moderates how quickly we break down calories and digest food, allowing us to process food and its nutrients more efficiently.

In the cardiovascular system, the ECS works to dilate blood vessels and weaken heart contractions, both of which reduce blood pressure and regulate heart rate. The ECS also affects the baroreflex, our body's built-in mechanism for maintaining even blood pressure.

In our endocrine system, a balanced ECS keeps disorders like diabetes, hypothyroidism, and hyperthyroidism at bay. The ECS regulates how we create and maintain bone cells, creating new skeletal cells when the body experiences bone damage.

Since the ECS is integral to every system in the human body, supporting its healthy function is essential, and we'll talk about that more specifically soon. Let's now take a closer look at how the ECS affects stress and pain, which are, in my own practice and teaching, the most crucial functions to understand at a chemical level.

THE ECS, STRESS, AND RESILIENCE

In the brain, stress is processed in the hypothalamus, pituitary gland, amygdala, prefrontal cortex, and hippocampus, all of which contain high concentrations of cannabinoid receptors. These, and the cannabinoids that bind to them, play a critical role in determining the level of threat a stress will pose, and then reacting to and processing the stress accordingly. Here's how this works.

When we experience stress, get nervous or fearful, our levels of cortisol, a stress hormone, go up. In response to that increase, the body creates more endocannabinoids. They move backward from postsynaptic neuron to presynaptic neuron, bind to the receptors there, and prevent the neurons from firing stress signals. That translates to the brain as less stress. So the brain signals for the production of less cortisol, bringing us back from off-balance, returning us to homeostasis. The cannabinoids are acting to lower "volume" on the noise of those signals.

The next time we encounter that same stress, or source of anxiety or fear, we produce even more cannabinoids and thus even less cortisol, even less of that noise. So our body is responding to that stress more efficiently and we are finding balance much more readily. In other words, we are becoming more resilient.

What's more, it's a compounding effect: the better your body is at handling one specific stressor, the better it becomes at understanding other stressors. The first time you speak in public, you might produce a ton of cortisol and be up all night beforehand. But after you finish the speech and it goes okay, and then you do it again and again, your ECS helps your body "know" that it doesn't need to produce that much cortisol, and over time you become less and less anxious and fearful. Throw yourself into another potentially uncomfortable situation, and guess what? Again, the ECS signals for less cortisol. Again, you're not nearly as scared or anxious.

THE ECS, PAIN, AND CONDITIONING

Pain is not efficient. More specifically, the imbalances and incongruities that lead to focal points of pressure that we perceive as pain or weakness force muscles, some organs, and some bodily systems to work harder than others, which results in an overall body inefficiency. Compensating for weak spots saps a whole lot of our energy.

That's what was going on with Tony Blauer. He had so many focal points of pain popping up all over his body that his entire system was working, like Whac-A-Mole, to tamp them down. As you'll know if you've ever tried it at a carnival, Whac-A-Mole is a real ordeal of a game. You think all you're doing is swinging your arm to hammer down the moles as they pop up, but in fact your entire body and mind are engaged in a state of throbbing anticipatory panic, and by the end, you are sweaty and spent.

An optimally functioning ECS regulates the transmission and reception of pain signals and thus keeps the pain (along with the anxiety of anticipated pain) under control. From peripheral nervous system to central nervous system, our pain circuits are abundant with endocannabinoids and receptors, the most important of which is anandamide. When produced and bound with a CB1 receptor, anandamide inhibits and reduces our perception of pain.

Also, as with stress, the ECS learns from its own response. Over time and exposure, it helps us to differentiate pain that is a real long-term threat from pain that is fleeting. So we learn to lean into the latter as a way of strengthening ourselves against the former.

WHEN THE SYSTEM DOESN'T WORK

Given how central the ECS is to all of our bodies' essential processes, it's no surprise that it's the key to healing from all of the common ailments that we explored earlier. It helped Josh Holland transcend the pain of intense spinal/posture retraining. It helped Seychelle Webster find a more optimal way of moving and then rebuild her body accordingly. The ECS is the mechanism that maintains our homeostasis amidst all of these physical and mental stresses and changes.

How does this vital omnipresent master balancer itself stay balanced? A healthy ECS produces enough cannabinoids to do its job well, all the time, for our entire lives. But like any other aspect of our health, it's a system that functions best when it is adequately and actively supported and nourished. If it isn't, the ECS can falter or fail us.

In some cases, the body isn't making enough cannabinoids, or their molecules are somehow defective. Sometimes there are not enough cannabinoid receptors in the body, or there are too many enzymes that break the endocannabinoids down before they can bind to a receptor. And sometimes there is just weak communication between the receptors and cannabinoids. All of these are indicators of clinical endocannabinoid deficiency syndrome (EDS), and while we don't yet know exactly what causes it (remember, ECS science is still in its infancy), it is most likely the result of damage from the environment, injury, or disease rather than genetic predisposition.

Research so far suggests that endocannabinoid deficiency may be a factor contributing to irritable bowel syndrome, recurring migraines, and fibromyalgia. According to Dr. Ethan Russo, who's been leading EDS research, these difficult-to-pinpoint disorders all have one thing in common: "(t)hey all involve a sort of hyper-sensitivity to pain . . . In the case of migraine it's headaches, but also painful stimuli such as noise and bright light. For irritable bowel it's an acute awareness of the gut and phenomena that normally don't hurt are quite painful to people with that condition, and with fibromyalgia, you've got a generalized increase in pain sensitivity on certain muscles or fibrous tissues may hurt to a great extent, but examining the tissue reveals no specific problem to explain it."

If you look at most of the other disorders that Russo suggests might be linked to EDS, you'll see clear links to functions that we know the ECS regulates. For example, we know that anandamide (the "bliss" cannabinoid) is good at helping us process and release harmful or nonuseful memories, which suggests that lower levels of anandamide might be a contributing factor of post-traumatic stress injuries. Other little-understood and treatment-resistant disorders or conditions Russo suggests might have a link to ECS deficiency include glaucoma, cystic fibrosis, infantile colic, and repetitive miscarriages.

The ECS can also be impaired by persistent stress, which reduces anandamide; lack of sleep, which can impede healthy stimulation of the CB1 receptors; and a diet heavy in trans fats, which can lead to excess inflammation and force the ECS into overdrive.

All of these elements of lifestyle can both lead to and reinforce an out-of-balance ECS.

KEEPING THE SYSTEM HEALTHY

Luckily, we have tools at our disposal to improve the functioning of our ECS and achieve a healthier homeostasis. Among them are the two protocols that we have already focused on in this book: Foundation Training (posture, strength, and breathing exercises) and heat/cold therapies. Beyond these, there are an infinite range of daily practices that can help us keep the ECS in balance, from meditation to yoga to walking and running. Even singing and dancing stimulate the ECS.

Central to all of these activities is deep, intentional breathing. As we talked about in the last chapter, a central goal of decompression breathing is to create more space for our body's systems to do their work—and that includes the ECS. The spine is the body's densest region of cannabinoid receptors—particularly at the very upper thoracic spine, at the cervical spine where the head meets the neck, and the lumbosacral region of the lower spine. (These are also the sites, you'll recall, of a great many significant nerve-plexus points.) So by increasing surface area with work like Foundation Training, you increase the efficacy and efficiency of those receptors. We also have CB2 receptors in our lungs. As we work on decompression breathing and posture and add heat, we are increasing the surface area exactly where these CB2 receptors are located.

Physical activity is essential to the optimal functioning of the ECS, too. Regular exercise stimulates the production of anandamide, which any of us who've experienced something like a runner's high know very well. But it doesn't have to be a strenuous endurance workout; bursts of intensity give you a huge squirt of anandamide, and low-impact activities like walking help, too. Higher levels of endocannabinoids in the blood can have long-term beneficial impacts on memory, mood, appetite, cognitive processing, and mental health. Recent science suggests that physical activity also enables increased expression of the cannabinoid receptor CB1 in the brain, which can improve memory and neural plasticity, create an antidepressant effect, and decrease neural inflammation. In one study, a three-minute isometric handgrip exercise led to an increase not just in anandamide and the endocannabinoid 2-AG, but also in lipids that regulate appetite and inflammation, and in the expression of CB1, resulting in noticeable pain relief.

The common principle in all of these activities, again, is frequent active adaptation. We're training ourselves to do something that at first feels unfamiliar, difficult, and even painful (emptying the mind, stretching a certain way, withstanding extreme heat), but with practice becomes noticeably easier. We are encouraging our endocannabinoid system to learn.

To underscore here: we are generating stress on purpose, with focused intention. By going *through* conflict as opposed to avoiding it, by working toward a goal—and bumping up against the physical, emotional, and creative strain that goes along with this—you're inoculating yourself against future stressors that will come your way, whether you like it or not. The ECS's work-to-reward system teaches the body that stress is a natural component of life, during which it needs to maintain itself.

I probably don't need to say much about avoiding trans fats and fast food. Suffice it to say: just as they're no good for the rest of the body, they're no good for the ECS. On the other hand, there are plenty of foods that actively stimulate our body's production of endocannabinoids, and I'll talk about those in the final chapter: a typical healthy human diet full of omega-3, omega-6, and omega-9 fatty acids.

Our bodies are intelligent builders. We take these molecules from what we eat and have found a way to use them to stimulate our own internal regulatory and reward mechanisms. That is our adaptation system at work.

Just as we can stimulate our body to create its own endocannabinoids, we also have at our disposal healthful exogenous cannabinoids: cannabinoids that come from outside the body but bind with the receptors in our body. Which brings us full circle: back to the amazing cannabis plant that sparked the discovery of this incredible bodily system. Among the hundred-plus cannabinoids found in cannabis, two of the most important of those are CBD and THC.

CANNABIS: AN INTRODUCTION

For so long, we have vilified and criminalized cannabis and used it carelessly. Now at last we are rediscovering it, destigmatizing it, exploring how it interacts with our minds and bodies. Since the cannabinoids we produce naturally are so essential to our health and well-being, it stands to reason that we should take a good hard look at what these externally produced cannabinoids can offer as well.

Cannabis has long been an integral component of my own health regimen. Over the past few years, it has become something I talk about openly with my long-term Foundation patients as well—as a tool for learning and training for them to explore. After all, cannabis is an incredibly effective means of stimulating our endogenous cannabinoid system, and that—alongside heat therapy and strength, posture, and breath work—is a core tenet of my philosophy of wellness.

That said, while I can confidently claim years of formal education and experience in human anatomy, treating pain, and physical training, I don't pretend to be a scientific expert on cannabis, just an experienced fan of the plant. I am a voracious investigator and researcher, and I passionately connect my learning with my own experience and practice. I am not, however, foolish enough to claim to have a prescription for everyone—about cannabis or anything else, for that matter. In this chapter, I will share what has worked for me and many of my patients, and what I have learned about the science behind it. Ultimately I encourage you to embrace your own cannabis education, to find your own way—or not—to integrate this plant into your journey toward health and wellness.

Before we dive in, a major caveat: I don't think anyone should start consuming cannabis until they are twenty years old unless it is medically prescribed for seizure or major anxiety disorders. Up until then, your brain is still actively developing, and marijuana could impede that process. It can decrease your motivation by making your body and mind expect pleasure too easily and passively, rather than cultivating a strong correlation between work and reward. You have almost a quarter of a century to *earn* your spot with pot!

So remember Mr. Mackey from *South Park*: "Drugs are bad, m'kay?"

For everyone over forty, my advice is precisely the opposite: you owe it to yourself to open your mind and give cannabis a legitimate shot. Now let's take a look at how trainer Josh Holland, whom we met in an earlier chapter, came to connect and reconnect with the plant.

Josh Holland, Celebrated Trainer

In high school, we couldn't drink soda during track season. This was a small town in Oklahoma and we were state champions, so if anybody saw you drinking soda, they're gonna jump all over you. So if there's a ban on soda, I'm definitely not going to drink alcohol, either. And you can't imagine the darkness around pot. You just don't do it. "That's gonna make you sterile, you're never gonna be able to have kids!" Mind you, my dad had been the chief of police and everybody knew him, so it was like: "The Holland brothers would never smoke weed." I didn't experience cannabis until I was twenty-four, after I'd graduated college. I had two experiences where nothing seemed to happen, then one horrible experience where I mixed it with alcohol and I thought, *Never again.*

Then, three years later, I tried edibles and it was nothing like before: in the middle of the day, not at night, and I was cleaning up my apartment. All of a sudden, I realized that I was able to hone in on what I was doing at the moment in this incredible way, to focus and get everything done. So I did it again the next time I was cleaning. Then I started doing research, learning more about cannabis. I was never a huge reader before then, but I challenged myself to read a book a week for a year, and I did it—easy. I had found something that allowed me to get rid of the noise. I dove into all the different strains, the way you consume it, the amount you consume . . . Instead of a party drug, I treated it like what it was: a medicine.

Josh's evolving relationship with cannabis is common to more people than I can count: friends, family members, colleagues, and patients of all kinds. In fact, it is a mirror for how our entire culture has been shifting. My own story with cannabis is not that different.

CANNABIS AND ME

Whereas I've relied on patient stories for the rest of this book, I am sharing mine here for a few reasons. It speaks powerfully to how cannabis can help us open up new doors in our lives. Also, when I called up patients to ask them to tell their own stories for this book, few of them were champing at the bit to talk about their cannabis use. This speaks, of course, to the enduring power of that stigma. By sharing my own story, I hope to encourage other people to open up as well, on their own terms. The continued legalization of cannabis in this country, as well as the increase in scientific research that will no doubt accompany this, is essential to destigmatization.

Remember: back in 2007, as I was finishing graduate school, I was diagnosed with degenerative joint disease in my back. "This is unstable and it's going to get worse and worse," doctors told me. "You're probably going to want to get fusion surgery pretty soon." They prescribed a strong painkiller/muscle relaxer, which was quite similar to what my dad had been offered by doctors for his back pain as I was growing up.

My dad wanted to avoid taking painkillers, but he did not have the tools we now have, so he would turn to them occasionally when back pain got unmanageable. These drugs tend to dissociate you, to make your whole body detach from feeling, and to inhibit your reflexes. So, for example, if you're about to fall over, you're just observing yourself, thinking, *I'm falling over*, instead of stopping yourself or bracing for impact. That disconnection is horrifically dangerous, particularly for the older people to whom these medications are often prescribed.

When I got that prescription, I was full of anxiety for other reasons—chiropractic school, failing my board exams—and the thought of adding a medication to the mix, especially one this strong, freaked me out. There I was, a big twenty-seven-year-old jock, lying on the floor when the pain hit, thinking, *Not again, not again! Why does this keep happening?!* I was equally afraid of the pain and the medication.

Then, during a heavy back spasm, I took the medication. On the plus side, it completely turned the spasm off for forty-eight hours. But there was an unfortunate side effect: everything else in me seemed to turn off, too. I couldn't go to school or drive; I couldn't coherently function. It wasn't just my body; my brain was in a fog, too. When the spasms were horrible, I took it a few more times and usually went right to sleep. I knew I needed a different solution.

That's when I turned to cannabis. I had used it before—for recreation, not medication. I was fully expecting to feel some dissociation as a side effect, as I had with the prescribed painkiller, but hopefully to a lesser degree.

In fact, I found that I was functioning *more* clearly. There was no brain fog at all, and I was not noticing my back as much, either. Not that the pain was turned off; I just wasn't scared of it. In fact, quite the opposite. Lying there, a little stoned, I wasn't asking, "Why me?" I was asking, "What *is* this?" I was *curious* about my pain. The feeling was not dissociation; it was association.

That is the best description I can come up with to describe my fourteen-year experience with cannabis, which continues to this day. It has made life so much more curious for me. The curiosity started with my back injury and evolved into questions about my mental and physical well-being more broadly. "Why do I wake up some days in a really bad mood for no reason? Maybe it's dietary? Maybe I'm not sleeping well enough?" I started actively looking for ways to improve myself, in places I hadn't looked before. THC and CBD were helping me connect dots, internally.

When I was twenty-seven, I was offered the incredible opportunity to be the strength coach and chiropractor/team doctor for the U.S. Men's Olympic Water Polo Team for the 2008 Beijing Olympics. It was an intense job: every morning I woke up at five-thirty to train and treat these athletes twice a day, six days a week for eleven months. At first I was terribly anxious, daunted by this amazing group of Olympiads. I wanted to do a good job but suffered from a severe case of impostor syndrome.

What nobody knew at the time, except for my girlfriend and some close friends, was this: I got through it with supplemental use of cannabis. I didn't need much, either. A couple of tokes before practice and I would relax, jump in the gym or even in the water with the guys, get playful and surprisingly creative. I was able to tune into what the team needed, more and more instinctively, and so the workouts became increasingly effective. The team went on to massive success.

In 2011, I was invited to do a TED talk, my first public speaking experience, and I was completely terrified. Backstage, going over what I wanted to say, I was sweating and shaking, my heart racing out of control. I had some pot with me and a chillum (a small glass pipe used for small doses of cannabis). But at the time, even after a few real successes with it, I still was on the fence about pot, its benefits versus its drawbacks, whether it was "good" or "bad" for me.

Then, when I finally made the call in my head, it felt so natural. Ten minutes after consuming (two small tokes), I felt as though my blood pressure dropped twenty points. I strolled up onstage and greeted the audience with a confident smile, like I was supposed to be there, like I was doing exactly what I was meant to do. I was able to meet them where they were, because cannabis met me where I was and gave me what I needed.

Going into that talk, I had had a rough idea of what I wanted to cover, the two patient stories that I would use. But when I started talking, the words and the order and the rhythms were all improvised. Cannabis had opened up a channel for me; it had taught me the feeling of flow. From then on, every time I teach, with or without cannabis, I have been able find that same feeling.

That talk catapulted my career. Two years later, I was traveling around the country teaching certification courses, and at the same time, studying for my third attempt at the chiropractic board exams, having failed twice before. On one level, it was a strained dynamic: teaching other doctors while unable to complete the same license myself. But unlike my previous experiences with the test, this time I used cannabis while studying as a readily available reward for work accomplished. It kept me focused and surprisingly driven.

Before I even left the exam, I knew I'd aced the test. Sure

enough, when my scores arrived, it turns out I had passed my boards with flying colors. That moment was the culmination of a years-long transformation, and from then on, I have not doubted the efficacy of cannabis for someone like me—not for a second.

A few qualifiers. I consume in sensible moderation—enough to make me loose, but no more than that, because I really don't like feeling stoned. I don't use alcohol or any other "unhealthy" substances. Not everybody's interactions with this plant are like mine, I know; we all have different brain chemistries and genetics.

But looking at my life before cannabis and after, I really can't compare the two. Back then, I was young and cocky, with less self-respect and an aggressive desire to prove myself, to intimidate people with my knowledge. Once I found pot, I became physically introspective with my injuries and mentally introspective with my thought patterns, sense of self, and connections to other people. I got curious about my profession, my entire existence, and my relationships. How can I learn from my patients? How can I reach out to someone struggling? How can I connect with my wife and remain a thoughtful father?

A BRIEF HISTORY OF A CRIMINALIZED MEDICINE

It is almost impossible for me to conceive of this plant that fits so seamlessly in our system, for the past century, being vilified and criminalized as a dangerous drug. It is anguishing that widely perpetuated falsehoods have left so many people in needless suffering. Yet, if we're ever to move beyond it, that's the history we have to reference and face.

Bookstores are filled with cleverly titled social histories of cannabis, and I can only scratch the surface here. For a deeper dive, there is a suggested reading list at the back of the book.

Three subspecies of cannabis have long been known and used for their mind-altering and medicinal properties: *Cannabis sativa*, *Cannabis indica*, and less common, *Cannabis ruderalis*. Then there's non-psychoactive cannabis, *Cannabis sativa L.*, known as hemp, grown and used to make all kinds of stuff, from fuel to food to clothing and shoes.

Cannabis originally evolved on the grassy steppes of the Tibetan plateau, possibly as long as 28 million years ago, and it is one of the plants that humans have grown and cultivated the longest. In ancient China, cannabis was used as a surgical anesthetic, and it was prescribed for malaria, fatigue, and rheumatism.

Over time, the plant spread via trade and nomadic cultures to Central Asia, into the Middle East, to Russia and Ukraine, Germany and Europe, across Africa, and, as early as the fifteenth century, to South and then North America. Throughout the nineteenth and early twentieth century United States, cannabis was a popular oral medication for pain, headaches, and spasticity, listed for years in the *United States Pharmacopoeia*.

While the usage of cannabis for health purposes has been a widespread and unbroken phenomenon in human history, the regulation and criminalization of cannabis was much more haphazard. Among notable historical prohibitions worldwide: Pope Innocent VIII denounced marijuana (and witchcraft) in 1484, and Napoleon banned his soldiers from using it after invading Egypt and Syria at the end of the eighteenth century. Throughout the 1800s, Britain tried and failed to ban cannabis in colonial India, an effort culminating in a study of cannabis that concluded, basically, that moderate habitual use of the drug was widespread and not at all harmful to individuals or society.

But in early twentieth century America, the knives really came out—first, from the nascent pharmaceutical industry itself. Until then, Americans had relied largely on homeopathic and herbal remedies, a homegrown tool kit that often included cannabis (for a time, one of the three medicines prescribed most). According to Dr. Rachel Knox, a specialist in cannabinoid medicine, the problems began with "two guys who really wanted to sell a lot of prescription drugs": tycoon/philanthropists Andrew Carnegie and John D. Rockefeller, who funded the 1910 Flexner Report, a study that advocated a sweeping industrialization of medical education. As Knox recounts:

[W]ith millions of dollars in their pocketbook, a document called the Flexner Report and the full force of state governments, American medical training was consolidated and standardized in accordance with pharmaceutical drug science to the exclusion of holistic care practices, natural substances and remedies and natural cures. And this created a system that made patentable pharmaceutical drugs that treated symptoms easy to sell, and that made natural holistic care and practices and unpatentable plant medicine like cannabis fringe, "quackery" and illegal.

As the century progressed, another force fed into the marginalization of cannabis, too: racism. When Mexican immigrants fled the 1910 Mexican Revolution for the southwestern United States, they brought cannabis, a popular recreational drug, which xenophobic white Americans saw as a symptom of their danger and degeneracy. That same stigma was aimed at other cannabis-using populations as well, from West Indians along the Gulf Coast to immigrant Indian agricultural workers in California to African Americans everywhere.

Then came the dogged fear-mongering of Harry Anslinger, the first commissioner of the Federal Bureau of Narcotics, who insisted that cannabis was the cause of "insanity, criminality, and death." With major assists from the hysteria of newspaper magnate William Randolph Hearst and a church-funded propaganda movie called *Reefer Madness*, anti-cannabis forces persuaded Congress to pass the Marihuana Tax Act of 1937, which criminalized cannabis possession nationwide and put the plant under the regulatory control of the Drug Enforcement Agency. In doing so, legislators ignored sustained objections by the American Medical Association and health-care practitioners who prescribed cannabis for medical usage. The anti-weed drumbeat reached its climax with the 1970 Controlled Substances Act, which classified marijuana as a Schedule 1 drug, the same category as heroin and LSD—meaning that it is easily addictive and abused, with no valid medical use.

Fortunately, science and popular opinion have been pushing back, harder and harder. The 1990s ushered in a tidal wave of de-criminalization, with state after state voting to allow possession and medicinal and recreational use of cannabis. Nevertheless, that Schedule 1 designation remains in effect to this day, arrests for cannabis possession persist at a breakneck pace, and an unconscionable number of men and women are behind bars for cannabis-related offenses.

The ongoing demonization of cannabis has been abetted by the pharmaceutical industry, which (correctly) sees the plant as a business threat and has lobbied against liberalization, just as oil and lumber industries oppose the increased use of hemp. But by now, rigorous scientific inquiry is bearing out what the homeopaths and naturopaths knew all along, and there is simply no getting around the plant's medicinal efficacy. No surprise, then, that Big Pharma—after years of fighting cannabis—is now eager to get in on the game, pouring money into synthetic CBD and THC.

Apart from millions of unjust incarcerations and a century of unnecessary mental and physical suffering, one of the most tragic results of America's crusade against cannabis is that research into the plant was severely stunted for so long. Once the government declared it a dangerous drug, any scientific study that might question or challenge that conclusion faced a huge uphill battle. Fortunately, society is catching up now, learning something new about this incredible plant every day. Here, let's talk about what scientific inquiry proves and suggests and what so many of us have learned from studying cannabis in our own lives.

HOW IT WORKS: THC

Earlier in this chapter, we talked about how to maintain and restore a healthy endocannabinoid system by nourishing the production of cannabinoids in our body—taking conscious control of our exercise, diet, and overall lifestyle. The introduction of exogenous cannabinoids, derived from the plant cannabis, is another way to do this. The cannabis plant contains about a hundred different cannabinoids, but we're going to talk about only the two most well-known ones, THC and CBD.

THC, which mostly comes from cannabis leaves and flowers, is psychoactive, meaning it affects the mind and perception. But if you consume cannabis raw, you're not going to feel much of anything. For THC to really work in the body, the outer ring of its molecular structure must be broken off, a process known as decarboxylation, which depends on time and/or heat: either by extended "curing" or by concentrated heating for at least 35 to 40 minutes at approximately 220°F.

In a lot of ways, THC is the exogenous counterpart to anandamide, the cannabinoid that our body produces on its own. Like anandamide, THC binds with the CB1 and CB2 receptors, but particularly and most importantly with the CB1 receptors in the central nervous system.

THC is a powerful reactive agent, highly concentrated in the cannabis bud and flowers, which is why we perceive its effects so quickly after consumption of even the tiniest amount: one hit and you feel that something's different. But even if it has been grown to be hyperconcentrated, up to 30 or 31 percent cannabinoids, the body can easily handle it in controlled doses.

The most efficient and effective way to deliver cannabis to the body is by smoking it: it absorbs much more rapidly (from lungs to brain in 20 to 30 seconds) and you can (and should) carefully control how much you take in. Contrast this with a gummy or a pill, which gives you a stronger and longer-lasting high, and because it can take over an hour to metabolize and be fully felt, can lead to overconsumption.

That widespread notion that smoking pot is as bad as smoking cigarettes has been debunked by recent science. While smoking tobacco is known to lead to lung cancer, smoking cannabis is not, and when cannabis is consumed responsibly (most studies use a joint as the daily dosage), you're unlikely to have any irritation or other ad-verse long-term effects on the lungs at all. If you're hacking up a lot of sputum or you get bronchitis, chances are you're either smoking way too much or also smoking tobacco. If you do need your daily cannabis dosage to be higher for medical reasons, you might want to vary smoking with another mode of intake.

After THC enters the body through the lungs, the lungs filter it rapidly through the entire bloodstream. The blood carries THC to every sensory system, organ, and tissue in the body. It is at this level, the level of organs throughout the body, that the somatosensory system exists. Remember, that's the system that controls the sen-sations of pain, body temperature, balance, vibration and pressure, and positioning and movement. Signals move from somatosensory receptors, synapse to synapse, to the central nervous system (brain), which interprets their activity and generates responses in the form of perceptions.

When THC enters this process, it works just like the canna-binoids we have in our bodies—backward and rebelliously across synaptic clefts, from postsynaptic receptor to presynaptic receptor. Here, THC binds with the presynaptic receptor and alters its capac-ity to send signals of sensation to the central nervous system. We'll talk about what specific bodily functions and processes THC affects in just a second.

HOW IT WORKS: CBD

CBD (or cannabidiol) comes from that other cannabis subspecies, *Cannabis sativa L.*, also known as hemp. It doesn't have the same perception-altering capability as THC, but it does have plenty of other usages—mainly to reduce pain, inflammation, and anxiety and aid with restful sleep. CBD works on its own, and as we'll see, it also works really well in conjunction with THC.

Unlike THC, CBD does not directly bind with the body's cannabinoid receptors, but rather, it stimulates their activity via other kinds of interactions with our ECS. It promotes the creation of the endogenous cannabinoid 2-AG, which we talked about earlier. It helps to sustain the potency of the other cannabinoid anandamide by blocking the activity of the enzyme that breaks anandamide down. CBD also binds with another super-important (non-cannabinoid) receptor in the body, TRPV1, which regulates pain, inflammation, and body temperature.

Through all of these processes, CBD helps our endocannabinoid system to work more effectively. That means it can be a great tool in our ongoing effort to achieve and improve homeostasis, to keep our bodies and minds functioning with more efficiency and resilience.

Not all methods of CBD intake, however, are the same. In the few years since its legalization in 2018, CBD has been all the rage, touted in any number of products, from oils and oral supplements to coffee, cookies, and lube, sold at drugstores and gas stations alike. An alarming number of these products have labels that inaccurately represent their actual CBD content, not to mention that they can contain harmful unlisted ingredients. Undoubtedly, many of them don't do anything at all.

So, as with everything, do your research and educate yourself before purchasing. Specifically, make sure you know how and where the hemp was cultivated, that the product has been independently tested for contaminants, and what its CBD concentration really is. If you don't have a specific cannabinoid prescription, I recommend a full spectrum product, one that includes a wide array of cannabinoids, so that you get the greatest benefit possible: the more cannabinoids, the more they can assist one another to help your body. But if you are getting tested for cannabis at work, make sure what you consume is free of THC.

Now let's get a bit more specific and talk about exactly what systems and processes these two cannabinoids can affect, individually and together. In my own cannabis education, this is where it all got super interesting to me, where I began to really see and feel the adaptive power of cannabis.

CBD AND THC: HOW THEY HELP

Earlier we talked about how endogenous cannabinoids (namely anandamide) affect all kinds of things, including our perception of pain. THC works the same way, but with much greater potency and thus greater effect. In a different way, CBD also affects pain. Not unlike how acupuncture is used as an anesthetic, CBD limits the transmission and translation of all kinds of pain, all over the body.

Neuropathic pain, created by disease or damage to our somatosensory system, is quite common and can be chronic and horribly debilitating. It can exist in the peripheral nervous system or the central nervous system or both. While neuropathic pain has been hard to treat with pharmaceuticals (we'll explore the problems with opioids in a second), there is an ever-growing body of evidence that cannabinoids, targeting the body's cannabinoid receptors, are effective. Studies have shown that the THC in inhaled cannabis produced profound relief in patients with cancer, diabetes, HIV, and trauma, those with chronic pain from spinal cord injury or disease, and sufferers of chronic pain caused by a compressed or inflamed spinal nerve. Recently, Canada approved both THC and CBD for treatment of neuropathic pain in multiple sclerosis. In a study involving 523 patients with HIV infections, 90 to 94 percent of the subjects using cannabis experienced improvement in muscle and neuropathic pain.

Cannabis is also dramatically effective in treating acute and chronic inflammation (our body's reaction to any number of conditions and illnesses), which is a common cause of the pain we feel. As an anti-inflammatory agent, THC is twice as potent as hydrocortisone and twenty times as powerful as aspirin. It inhibits PGE2 synthesis to diminish the inflammation common to rheumatoid arthritis and osteoarthritis, and decreases blood platelet aggregation that can cause clotting.

THC is also a potent antioxidant and antispasmodic agent, which, along with CBD, is known to impede the progress of multiple sclerosis and help patients with Huntington's disease. It also combats Alzheimer's by blocking harmful plaque formation.

Like THC, CBD alleviates pain, inflammation, and spasms on its own. But it doesn't alter perception, which is why some people prefer it. CBD works with and even modulates THC, reducing some of THC's psychoactive effects, as well as symptoms like lethargy, a racing heart, and anxiety, and that makes THC consumption more tolerable. (This is known as the entourage effect.) Both THC and CBD work to lessen nausea, significantly one of the most impairing side effects of cancer treatment. As I've seen in many people, THC prevents shaking and other symptoms of Parkinson's (with an assist from CBD to rest their system). In 2018, the FDA approved the very first cannabis-derived drug ever in the United States, a CBD-based medication proven to control epileptic seizures.

People are taking CBD for more and more common reasons these days, and there is plenty of scientific and anecdotal evidence of its effectiveness. Most of us probably know people who swear by CBD for restful sleep, to prevent insomnia, and/or to reduce generalized anxiety. Doctors of all kinds are prescribing CBD for conditions like musculoskeletal pain and are reporting great success. In the realm of cardiovascular health, CBD is known to reduce blood pressure, heart rate, inflammation, and cell death related to heart disease. On an overall level, the science of CBD is in its infancy, but what we do know so far is truly promising.

CANNABINOIDS VERSUS OPIOIDS

While we're focusing on cannabis and pain management, I think it's worth taking a closer look at the main "competitor" in this realm: opioids. Superficially, cannabinoids and opioids have a lot of similarities. Both boast a long, rich history of recreational and homeopathic medicinal use. They are both naturally produced in the body and also administered exogenously, and they react with receptors to alter bodily functions. Both are psychoactive, meaning they alter the function of the central nervous system; and both produce a lot of the same kinds of feelings, including euphoria. Also, both are really effective in lessening the feeling of pain.

But it's opioids that have been far more commonly embraced by the pharmaceutical and medical industry as the go-to source for pain management. I don't have to tell you about the catastrophe of overprescribing and overusing that has ensued as a result. Opioids are far more addictive than cannabinoids, and in our ongoing opioid crisis, millions of people have overdosed and died, many of them very young. Even with the liberalization of public policy around cannabis, you won't see anyone overdosing on it.

A major reason for this is concentration. In fact, this is the biggest difference between opioids and cannabinoids. Opioids in and of themselves are not dangerous to the human body, but *concentrated* opioids are, and that's the form they often come in. In a period of a couple hundred years, opium has morphed from a natural, harmless pleasure derived from the poppy plant to drugs with a concentration that can literally kill you.

On a broader, more essential level, I think there's another key difference between the two systems. The opioid system is largely about a specific kind of pain relief: numbing. That means shutting down or dissociating not just from sensation, but from activity, life in general. The cannabinoid system is more inherently active; it's about pleasure, belonging in and engaging with life, connecting with the world around you. Chemically speaking, opioids are about checking out. Cannabinoids are about checking in.

Increasingly, the medical community is embracing cannabis as a safer and less addictive source of chronic pain relief. Doctors are weaning opioid-addicted patients slowly off their Vicodin or Oxy-Contin and introducing them to THC and CBD, and reports from patients are overwhelmingly positive.

THE MIND: CANNABIS, CURIOSITY, AND CREATIVITY

Remember Seychelle Webster, the stand-up paddleboarding champion who injured her neck? She, too, is a cannabis proponent and eagerly volunteered the fact, in order to combat stigma and help other athletes suffering through injuries. "Cannabis has been a big part of my healing process," she says. "I am a proponent of plant medicine."

You might assume that Seychelle uses cannabis primarily for treating her pain. In fact, for her, it's so much more. She uses CBD for occasional bouts of tension and acute anxiety, and almost every night before going to bed to sleep more restfully. In addition to that, she uses THC almost daily for different reasons entirely.

> THC I use most days as my "off switch" for work and my "on switch" for creativity. So it's usually an afternoon/after work/relax/go for a walk on the beach and let my mind be free time. If I don't use THC, I find it difficult to stop working/turn off my work/go-go-go mind. It helps me feel more creative.

Seychelle is very much onto something, and her experience with cannabis as an activator of creativity is shared by many people, me included. To me, pot has been the grandest motivator that I have ever had. It lets me move through a process, from imagining to executing to finishing. The stereotypical lazy pothead thing has never been my own experience.

As I mentioned up front, cannabis lets me tune into my anatomy and physicality like nothing else I've tried. It lets me have a focused, open, and productive internal dialogue with my body, head to toe. In a very real sense, that's because cannabis helps me turn a certain unproductive part of my mind off. The neurotransmitter glutamate is very excitatory, and it's often responsible for mental rumination or spinning thoughts, which waste so much energy. The cannabinoids in an indica-heavy strain of pot will disrupt that process, shifting CB receptors from mental sensation to peripheral sensation. A lot of people call this "couch lock" because it makes your limbs heavy, but it's really just an increased sensation: feeling the weight of your limbs in a way you usually don't. Cannabis shifts our focus from mind to body, which is one of the most important things we can do: get out of our heads. It moves our energy from useless mental rumination and pushes it outward, into our body and movement.

Many people in my life—athletes, musicians, family members, scientists, and doctors—look at cannabis in a positive way and have experienced its benefits. Think of Josh Holland, who, thanks to cannabis, challenged himself to read a book every week for a year. Or how about these words from one of the most successful pot smokers in recent history, Apple founder Steve Jobs: "The best way I could describe the effect of the marijuana and hashish is that it would make me immediately relaxed and creative." Or comedian and long-time cannabis user George Carlin, who once told Jon Stewart that he kept a joint on him only for special moments where he needed an extra creative burst: "I hardly touch it, maybe once a month, but when I'm writing something perfectly sober, eight or nine pages. The next day . . . one hit, and it's *punch-up time.*" Common to all of these experiences is a sense of unlocking something that may have been closed off before: opening up to a new awareness of your own potential for growth and change.

In terms of scientific proof for this phenomenon, we do know that cannabis intake increases blood flow to all the same parts of the brain associated with creativity, specifically those that create sensations of reward and happiness. During the past ten years, there have been quite a few limited studies looking at the relationship between cannabis and creativity. One from 2012 seems especially relevant. It explored connections between cannabis and divergent thought, often viewed as a measure of creativity: the ability to respond to a problem in a range of ways, to answer open-ended questions and generate unique solutions. By contrast, convergent thinking involves looking for and channeling knowledge into one, right answer. The study measured divergent thinking via two groups of participants' ability to say as many words starting with a *b* or an *m* as possible in sixty seconds, and found a decisive correlation: after cannabis consumption, the "low creative" group's ability to think divergently increased dramatically, right up to the level of the "high creative" group. Another 2010 study found a correlation between cannabis consumption and increased semantic hyperpriming—coming up with uncommon or unpredictable connections between words that are only loosely related.

Not all studies, however, point in the same direction. Another experiment found that high-concentration THC impaired divergent thinking in regular cannabis users. Other studies have found little in the way of linkages at all. Finally, not to be too much of a downer, but both of the studies mentioned in the above paragraph looked at and found some relationship between heavy cannabis use and increased schizotypy, a collection of symptoms running the gamut from mild dissociation to schizophrenia and psychosis. So, just to reiterate all of my caveats from before: the risks of cannabis are real, there's a lot we don't know, and everybody responds differently. Educate yourself as fully as you can.

A frequent but unanswered question in much of this research is whether cannabis users are, personality-wise, predisposed to creativity and open-ended thinking to begin with. This would suggest that cannabis in fact may be taking us where we already were headed. I for one don't see this as a negative conjecture. In fact, it seems quite reasonable, and it pretty much sums up my own understanding and experience.

For the past fourteen years, I have been moving toward a more open-minded, unorthodox, and creative approach to the human body. Cannabinoids, through their stimulus-response adaptive system, have been helping me in that process: responding to my thrill of exploration, enabling me to push beyond my comfort zone and process what I have found there. On a physical level, cannabis helps me adapt my body further and further in the direction I am taking it, toward greater health and efficiency.

THE BODY: CANNABIS AND EXERCISE

While my expertise is limited to Foundation Training, I do try to get every patient I've ever interacted with safely off as many unnecessary pharmaceuticals as possible, to the best of my ability, through strength, movement, and breath work, heat therapy, and an ever-evolving collection of other protocols that I find valuable. I often share with them my own experience with cannabis as well. I encourage their curiosity about the plant, and if it feels right, I suggest that my patients give it a shot.

When does it "feel right"? It's always with people who I see have already taken the initiative in their training and wellness, who actively seek care and are ready to do the work themselves to receive the benefits of that care. They don't want to let their immediate physical detriment become their ultimate detriment. They don't want to be a patient who suffers Alzheimer's or multiple sclerosis and dies from it, or a patient who ends up having a leg amputated because peripheral neuralgia and neuropathy are so extreme. They aren't passive folks looking for a miracle, either. Rather, more often than not, they are active current or former athletes that just want to live the lives they love.

Every one of them gets the same thing, which is a steady amount of Foundation Training, as prescribed, for the rest of their lives. Breathing is another ingredient. Sauna is another ingredient. At times, so is cannabis. With all of these ingredients, based on what works for and connects with the patient themselves, we create all kinds of different recipes.

For those of you who have bought into the stereotype of the couch-potato stoner, using cannabis in conjunction with physical exercise might seem bizarre or impossible. But I know many high-performing athletes who swear by it during training, especially off-season training. In fact, studies have shown that in the United States, cannabis users are far less likely to be obese than nonusers. Let that sink in.

In one survey just last year, a Colorado social psychologist named Angela Bryan found that a vast majority of cannabis users—4 out of 5 of the 600 she questioned—reported consuming cannabis just before or after training. Those that added cannabis to their regimen spent longer exercising than those who didn't.

Most who added cannabis to their regimen said it made exercising more fun, which Bryan suggests has a chemical reason. You've probably heard of the runner's high, the euphoria you suddenly achieve at a certain point during a workout. That's often been attributed to our opioid system, pleasure-inducing endorphins activating opioid receptors. But what about the "bliss" molecule, the endocannabinoid anandamide? That produces euphoria, too. Like Bryan, I'm inclined to think that runner's high may in fact come from the endocannabinoid system, which means that THC can help activate it. While this is not yet scientifically proven, Bryan points to another reason for cannabis-induced exercise pleasure that resonates deeply with what I've learned from my patients and my own body. "If something feels good, you're going to want to do it again."

Cannabis isn't for every kind of training, of course. It definitely does not enhance performance for certain exercises. Rather, it enhances mechanics and somatosensation, and should be used during the days that you're doing gentle cardio, range-of-motion training, breath work training, and modest strength training. If you're not doing those things before you bring cannabis in, you should bring those things in first and then eventually do them together.

For pre-workout preparation, I recommend starting out with CBD alone, without mind-altering THC. CBD primes the efficiency of that glutamate and GABA cycle I mentioned earlier. It calms mental rumination and anxiety nicely, helps increase blood flow through the whole body, and helps the brain and body to connect a little bit more. This keeps you from drifting off, keeping you focused, with your body in a "ready to adapt" state. You're telling your body: "We're going to train."

When you start to exercise, whether you have smoked a CBD joint or taken a CBD tincture or edible, you're not going to feel dramatically different, other than a bit more energetic. But as you proceed, especially with exercise like cardio, you very likely *will* notice increased focus and clarity, and surprisingly *sustained* energy.

If you add THC to the mix, the cardio might be more fun, but it likely won't be faster. You might enjoy the feeling of lifting and training more, but you're probably going to want to take your weight load down 20 to 30 percent to reserve extra mental energy for somatosensation. That process has a very real caloric demand, too. In other words: max lift and max sensation do not go together.

Post-workout, no matter what your routine, taking THC and CBD later in the day gives you a more restful evening and a deeper sleep. In terms of recovery, an integral part of any training, THC and CBD are both effective at treating post-workout pains and soreness.

Even having said all this, I know it might still seem scary or "wrong" to some of you to use cannabis and exercise together. Before you try it, it will help to open yourself up to it mentally, as much as possible. Talk about it with those you trust. If you do find yourself opening up to the idea, start small and slow. Let yourself feel this new experience with as much focus and curiosity as possible.

WHAT TO TAKE AND HOW TO TAKE IT

If you're new to cannabis, it can feel hard or overwhelming to find the right way in. If you're a long-term casual cannabis user, you might not be so tuned into the subtle but crucial chemical specifics of what you're consuming or the ways that the cannabis market has changed and become more refined. So I'd like to share some broad insights and recommendations on usage, based on what I've seen in my own and my patients' experiences.

I always recommend that people start off with a mixed CBD/ THC strain. As I mentioned earlier, CBD has a nice benefit of calming down the psychoactive effect of THC, so it gives you kind of a slide-in, if you're not used to it. Some of these higher CBD

NOURISHING THE ENDOCANNABINOID SYSTEM 135

strains include Harlequin, Cannatonic, and Charlotte's Web, which is probably the most notable CBD strain available. Those are all very relaxing, but they don't drain your energy at all. They give you energy and clarity. They're great for work or for running, biking, or swimming laps; with these types of exercise, you experience a wonderful mental/physical connection.

I have two personal favorites. One is Sour Diesel, which I use to train my understanding of the tensions felt throughout my movements. It stimulates the whole process. When I need to be creative, to think deeply, I usually like to have Jack Herer, a strain named after one of the primary activists for the legalization of medical pot back in the day. The Jack Herer strain is really good sativa, incredible for creative thought processing, and if you're going through trouble—in a relationship, in a work situation—it gets you asking why; it gives you the opportunity to feel what's really going wrong.

THC concentration is key. A lot of people have made the mistake of starting with a sativa that has too much THC, which can result in mind-spinning and anxiety. This can turn you off cannabis. I suspect that's what happened when Josh had such a bad experience with pot in his early years. I always recommend to people just starting out: nothing above 17 percent THC for your first year. The next year, stay below 22 percent. The next year, stay below 25 percent. If you do that, you're far less likely to have an uncomfortable experience with cannabis.

Suppose during the first year or so that your body is registering this new plant and sensation, you overstimulate every time. Then you're going to feel really weird, and not in a good way. It would be as if when you first started drinking alcohol, all you did was get extremely drunk every time. If you go too heavy, too hard, you're not going to enjoy it, and it's not going to work the same. You don't want to drown the endocannabinoid system in stimulation; you simply want to stimulate it.

Then there's the question of how you should consume the cannabis. As I've said before, smoking is the method I prefer and recommend, for a variety of reasons: it's purer (less likely to contain additives and contaminants) and more immediately effective and you can control the dosage much more effectively.

There is of course a whole booming industry of edibles, and I can't say I'm a big fan. It's basically a whole marketplace of sweets, desserts, and crappy ingredients. Here we have this magical plant, this sensational, extraordinary thing that has adapted perfectly to fit into our systems, and we screw it up with gummy bears and pretzels. I'm looking forward to a larger, healthier world of edibles, but we're not there yet.

You should avoid anything flavored or with additives—flavored vapes, blunts in tobacco wraps with all kinds of chemicals. The goal is, again, to be as pure as you can be.

In sharing my own experience with and insights into cannabis, based on what I know and what I've learned from so many patients, I hope to open up more opportunities for people to talk and think, to explore and share the possibilities of this long-misunderstood substance. Right now, I'm fortunate to be part of a community that's unusually free and open about pot in our lives, and I realize that a lot of people are not in my position. In many places, legality issues and cultural stigma still make this kind of conversation impossible, uncomfortable, and/or dangerous.

It is my hope that we're nearing the end of this darkness. I'm grateful to those who have pioneered the way to get us this far in terms of cultural and medical acceptance, and I'm thrilled that more and more people are shining a light toward a better future. Across the world, every day, I hear about another expert in health or medicine, another athlete or artist or entrepreneur proudly declaring that cannabis is an integral component of their wellness tool kit, and I smile.

Let's wrap up with a return to one of those people, Josh Holland, the son of a chief of police from Oklahoma who, thanks to cannabis, became a voracious reader and a more active investigator of his own body. Josh is also a trainer, and as part of that job, he has come to share his experience and thinking on cannabis with his clients.

I use CBD every day with clients that are dealing with pain, and then that opens up the idea of going beyond that, into this whole world of plant medicine and the ECS. We talk amounts and strains and when and how it works to consume. When they start understanding that hey, we all have this endocannabinoid system that can be plugged into—that's when they really get it. We have this system in our body there—it's there. You can either deny it or you can work with it.

CHAPTER 5

Putting It All Together

Jessie Salas, Foundation Training
program director and lead instructor

When I left the fire service after sixteen years, I didn't realize how much I needed a structure. When you leave those guys that you've gone through all this intense life-and-death stuff with . . . That bond is different than most, and so when you leave that, mentally it affects you. You feel lost. When I had those moments, I started to realize: "Okay, I need some kind of routine." I needed to develop a new structure for myself.

As far as life changes go, Jessie's transition out of firefighting was pretty dramatic. It wasn't just a career shift; it was a transformation of his sense of purpose. It was about healing from physical and emotional injury and creating a new definition of wellness and balance that was all his own.

I consider myself lucky to be an ongoing witness to Jessie's adaptations. And while not all of my friends or patients have undergone such major shifts, many of them seem to be approaching big turning points in their lives, brought on by injury, stress, or unhappiness, sometimes all of the above.

But it's not the pain or trauma that defines the turning point; it's how they respond to it, how they adapt to it. It's Patti Sheaff, finding a way to continue doing what she loves. Or Tony Blauer, taking control of his training, challenging himself to run through pain. It's Seychelle Webster, facing a shattered career, then rethinking how her body moves and becoming stronger than ever. Or Evan Halquist, figuring out how to do his job more effectively and safely and helping spread the word to his fellow firefighters. In all of their stories, the pain is just the beginning, the thing that gets the exciting journey of change started.

In this section, we'll explore what that journey looks and feels like on a daily basis. We'll hear from patients, in their own words, about how they have incorporated the ideas in this book to live the lives they want. First, let's look back at the various protocols we've covered and spotlight some of the features they share. As you'll see, they work together to tell a much bigger story.

UNDERSTANDING AND TRANSLATING SENSATIONS

The basis of everything I teach, every practice and protocol, is understanding and translating sensations. That's the first crucial step in taking control of and being accountable for our own self-care: getting in touch with what we feel, being curious about it, instead of fearful. We can harness that curiosity to actively adapt and eventually become resilient. In order to do that, we have to understand that pain is a signal, an opportunity to learn. It's crucial to understand the "bigger story" the pain is telling us: how it connects with the overall ecosystem of our bodies; how it connects to our habitual behaviors or patterns of movement. More often than not, that involves tuning into the relationship between physical pain and what's going on in our minds, our emotions, and our lives more generally.

Stimulating the mind and body through the introduction of controlled stress is what brings about positive change. Becoming aware of our body positions and movements and working to subtly correct them; being aware of our breath and consciously engaging with it; sauna bathing to challenge our body and minds; stimulating our miraculous endocannabinoid system in order to facilitate the active adaptation process. These methods work together to help us meet all the challenges we face in life head-on.

SYNERGISTIC RESULTS

Active adaptation is about individual improvement in movement, posture, pain management, and stress response, but it's bigger than that, too. The feeling of reward we derive from the process itself is something that we can consciously apply more broadly across all aspects of our life. The better we get in one protocol or area, the better we get elsewhere, too.

Think of those ten extra minutes of anxiety that you push through in the sauna. After you teach yourself that you can handle it, you can apply that lesson to holding a difficult Foundation pose for another minute, climbing those few extra meters to a summit, or having an emotionally fraught but important conversation with a loved one. In all these situations, you're making an active decision to confront challenges with a level head.

Remember what Tony Blauer taught himself about pain? He felt, on his own terms, the difference between useful, adaptive pain and "harmful" pain, and over time, got better and better at avoiding/minimizing the latter, but working with the former. That's a skill we can apply to any kind of exercise, but also to management of any kind of pain, including emotional distress. Rather than looking for a quick fix from elsewhere (a doctor or pill), which leads to complacency and dependency, we work to get *ourselves* better, bit by bit. By listening to, looking at, and learning from pain, we take charge of it. And again there's that synergy: active adaptation to pain specifically encourages deeper body and mind awareness more broadly, and those become "muscles" we flex with all kinds of stimuli and experiences.

FOOD IS THE FUEL

Adaptation and change require energy, and the way we fuel our body is through food. I want to be clear that I am not a nutritionist, and faced with the wildly divergent and ever-changing diet advice emerging from the wellness industry and the scientific community, I'm not going to go into great detail. I am not a vegetarian or a vegan, but I do believe that with the proper research, you can provide your body with everything it requires following those dietary guidelines. I think of diet as purely a function of making sure your body has the right nutrients, those required for healthy, efficient adaptation. I know what works for me and what seems logical given how the body functions.

The most basic advice I can offer is to eat like an adult. What we eat has a huge effect on us, mentally and physically. How could it not? If you want pain relief, if you want to continue to be able to do the things that you enjoy, be responsible when it comes to food. If you eat the wrong things, you are wasting energy. Bad food disrupts our body's natural processes, forcing us to expend energy metabolizing something it didn't want in the first place. Good food provides clean energy that fuels our body, enabling effective communication among its parts.

Here are some very general tips that you've likely heard before. I've found them useful in my life and in the lives of my patients. Actively making better food choices, giving your body clean sources of energy, and staying properly hydrated makes all adaptive processes easier and more efficient.

Don't eat processed food. We should all know this by now. Food far removed from its natural source or filled with chemicals, preservatives, or growth hormones is in general not good for you. It's as simple as that.

Make sure you are getting the full spectrum of omega fatty acids. Fatty acids are important for maintaining your brain and digestive health, guarding against inflammation, beefing up your immune system, and providing your body with the fuel it requires to function optimally. Certain fatty acids stimulate endocannabinoids (particularly anandamide and 2-AG), which can, if under the right stress conditions, engage the ECS and trigger the adaptive response. However we decide to stress our system—exercise, heat, cold, meditation, hyperventilation—our body won't learn from it if we don't have enough fatty acids to work with. Avocados, avocado oil, sunflower seeds, nuts, flaxseed oil, real dark chocolate, grass-fed beef, fish, healthy dark meat poultry—there are numerous sources for omega fatty acids, and I encourage you to research them and make choices consistent with your lifestyle.

COMPLEMENTARY MODALITIES

There are other modalities that I find useful in maintaining balance, but since many books have been written on each topic, I will refrain from going into much detail. Again, I encourage you to do some research and try things out. Meditation is helpful, in whatever form you find comfortable. Remember how much energy rumination requires? If you're solving problems, that's energy well spent. If you are just obsessively having anxious thoughts, that's a waste. Learning to quiet your mind, even for just a few minutes a day, is invaluable. It reduces stress and helps you keep things in perspective. I mostly just do it when I'm sitting in the sauna, focusing on my breath, and trying to clear my mind.

I also find mantras instructive. When I'm feeling overwhelmed or agitated, I repeat to myself, "I have room for all of this and more." I've found it especially useful when it comes to pain management. Often in my life I've felt defeated by pain, like I just can't handle not being able to do what I want to do. This mantra lets me know that I'm going to be all right, that I'm not even near my capacity. It helps with interpersonal issues, work issues, just about everything. It reminds me that I am more resilient than I know.

The other phrase I find myself repeating is "Don't let discomfort doom you." Almost every poor decision I have made in my life was at a time of discomfort—when I was either stressed out or in pain. It's important to know when you should just be still and *not* make a choice. Accept where you are and see where it takes you. Don't let pain lead you into unnecessary surgery. Don't let a frustrating moment in your workplace compel you to do something rash. Get to a place where you can make a better decision, when you feel strong and healthy and stable.

COMING INTO BALANCE

But beyond each individual stress-response experience, the homeostasis it helps maintain has a greater purpose: achieving the most efficient output, the most efficient rest, the most efficient relationship, the most efficient life. And *efficient* also means *effective*—creating the most fruitful outcomes, making the biggest differences, not just in your own mind and body, but in the community around you, the people, animals, and nature that you interact with. In the presence of good self-care, there is a positive and compounding feedback loop.

Think about starting a new creative project. The more actively you envision and define your end results, the more actively you form the patterns of your work, the more productive and successful the project will be. Or think about being in a chronically frustrating work environment—you have complacently adapted into a state of just kind of muddling through it. Whether you can feel it or not, that condition takes a lot of unconscious energy to sustain, which is a waste, plain and simple. But the more you open up to the challenge of changing the environment—by talking and listening to coworkers, by reconnecting with your collective potential—the more energy you have to keep the change happening. And by actively nourishing one aspect in your life, you give yourself more drive to apply that same adaptive power elsewhere: making new friends, reaching out to people in need, thinking beyond yourself.

IT'S JUST ROUTINE

I hope while reading this book, you have gotten to know a few of the people whose lives have changed due to some of the principles we've explored. But the most important thing for me to emphasize is the ways they've changed how I think about what I do. They have, each in their own way, pushed me to make connections, explore possibilities, and broaden my definition of what it means to be healthy. Some, like Jessie, Alli, and Evan, have become integral parts of Foundation Training; others, like Seychelle, I've never even met in person. But they have each helped push the work we do further. I've asked them to provide a brief summary of their daily routines. If they look intimidating, keep in mind they have all, at this point, been practicing these modalities for years. And keep in mind, too, that when he started, Tony Blauer could hold Foundation positions for only a few seconds! Wherever you are is the place to begin. With every engagement, your mind and body will adapt and improve, taking you exactly where you want to go.

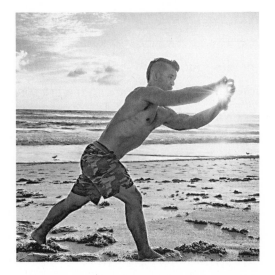

Jessie Salas

I start every morning with Wim Hof breathing, which is hyperoxygenation. It elicits adrenaline and wakes me up. I played with various breathing practices; they'd put me back to sleep. So I do a round of Wim Hof and I focus on gratitude, basically going through a laundry list of everything I have to be thankful for. When I transition from that, I generally would go into free-dive breathing (belly breathing) and focus on intent. What do I want to do for the day? What am I trying to achieve? What are my goals? And then I just go into breath of fire (rapid, forceful exhalations through the nose) and focus on things that make me happy. Once I am done with that, I do my Foundation Training. I start very gently, twenty seconds of work, ten seconds of rest. I'll do a supine decompression and then just flip-flop a couple different exercises. Then I basically go into journaling, just writing out notes and what my plan is for the day, structuring it. And I found, for me, it allowed my brain to, at the minimum, feel like,

"Look at how much I've achieved at the start of my day, and it's just started." It sets the tone for the day.

When I'm on the road, my routine can go out the window. I fall behind; I have setbacks. After leaving the fire service, I began wondering if I'd made the right decision. I'd find my brain going into this anxious, panicked, angry, or unsatisfied state. And it wasn't until I realized that I had stopped doing my routine, stopped setting intentions, that I understood how to fix it. When I do my routine, life is good; I have a clear path of what I'm working on, where I'm going, and what I want.

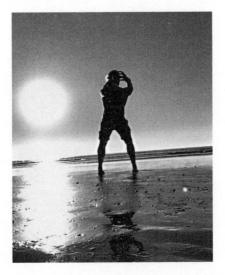

Tony Blauer

One of the most important things I learned from Eric is that it doesn't take a lot to start making changes. Every day, usually when I wake up and before I go to sleep, I do some sort of breathing meditation. This varies from conventional box breathing (just taking slow, deep breaths) to Wim Hof to some other breathing technique. I've discovered a few apps that I like a lot. Generally, anything that just makes you focus on your breathing is very helpful. I do a founder every morning while I'm brushing my teeth, and a Foundation routine every night before I go to bed. Often, during the day, I'll just do short poses or stretches if I feel like I need to. To de-stress and detoxify, I try to take a sauna at least three times a week. I'm still training and teaching five times a week, so I get plenty of cardio, but I also make sure to take a walk every day. I eat as clean and healthy as I can, and take vitamin D and a good fish oil.

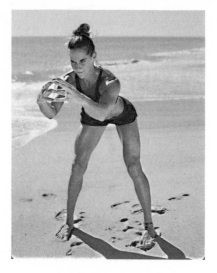

Seychelle Webster

I wake up an hour and a half before sunrise and spend 45 minutes either meditating or journaling. I drink a lot of water and have breakfast and coffee early, so I have a full meal digested before my morning training session. I walk across the street to see the sunrise, standing near enough to the water's edge so that the waves wash over my feet. I do a few founders and body traces and rotations. I like to catch the sun as it rises in my sphere of tension.

Typically, I do a 75- to 90-minute training session in the morning, paddling or strength training, and then eat again before starting work. I sneak some FT techniques in most things that I do: paddle warm-ups, rotations, and hinging with core stabilization. And during strength warm-ups and squats, I'm always aware of my cervical and thoracic spine positions, making sure I'm positioning myself correctly and activating the right muscles. At this point, Foundation Training is so blended in with how I move my body throughout the day that it is hard to separate out what I do specifically that is FT.

I use CBD for acute anxiety or tension during the day. Not every day, just as needed. I use it almost daily before going to bed to aid in more restful sleeping. THC I use most days as my "off switch" for work and my "on switch" for creativity. So it's usually an afternoon/after work/relax/go for a walk on the beach and let my mind be free time. If I don't use THC, I find it difficult to stop working/turn off my work/go-go-go mind. It helps me feel more creative. From time to time, I will use edibles as a sleep aid. I have been experimenting and working on optimizing my sleep recently and I have found that CBD works better for more restful sleep. Cannabis has been a big part of my healing process. I am a proponent of plant medicine. I am a mostly plant-based eater. I was vegan for fifteen years. Now I am technically vegetarian. I am usually in bed around 8:15 and asleep around 9:00 P.M. I do not set an alarm. I have such a habit of rising early that I let my body do so naturally.

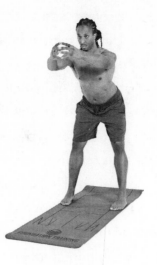

Josh Holland

In the morning, I make sure to soak up as much sun/light as possible and then go into some movement and stretching in the form of The Five Tibetan Rites. Then I usually practice some form of meditation and breath work. After that, I eventually make my special coffee and begin preparing to tackle the day.

As far as meals go, I practice intermittent fasting each day [fasting for 16 hours; restricting eating period to 8 hours], which takes the pressure off always having to decide what to eat from meal to meal.

Ultimately, I feel that quality awareness, rest, consumption, activeness, and exercise make up the key ingredients to optimal health and wellness.

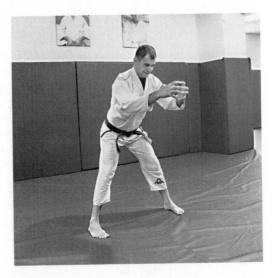

Jackson Fortunato

My workout routine daily is 20 to 25 minutes on the air assault bike, which is what really kicks my cardio in, followed by full-body exercises, usually push-ups, then 5 minutes of Foundation Training (founder and lunges with hip rotation). I usually do this workout at 9:00 A.M. after dropping the kids at school or after I finish my morning jiujitsu classes. I'm not doing any breath work at the moment, but I want to go back to it. When I do it, it's a 15-minute session with a guided audio from Wim Hof.

I have been taking only cold showers for nearly two years. I also do an ice bath immersion once a day for 3 minutes. After that, I do 3 to 5 minutes of Foundation work. I feel my body moving constantly using the FT principles—hip hinges and anchoring are part of my daily movements.

I do not follow any particular diet, because I don't believe in diets. I was vegan for approximately seven years, but then I realized that being vegan can also be unhealthy. I do eat a little of everything, but basically two meals a day, sometimes three.

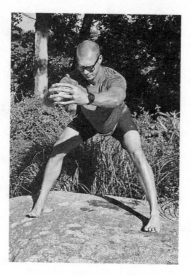

Erik Antonson

I do breath work to improve my heart rate variability before I catch waves. I find it sets me in the right place as I'm paddling in. And then again after each run to calm down. Foiling (riding a surfboard with a foil attached instead of a fin) is like a series of 800-meter sprints.

When we're in Connecticut, I hit the sauna almost every day, but in Florida we don't have one, so I'll do hot baths every few days. I hit the infrared sauna a couple times a week.

I do Foundation exercises before I surf, and every night. I've gotten my routine down to about 5 minutes for each session. If I get to a bad place for my back, I'll do longer workouts. Lots of decompression breathing throughout the day.

Diet: collagen protein, whey protein, liposomal supplement, vitamin C, vitamin D, NAD+, CocoaVia.

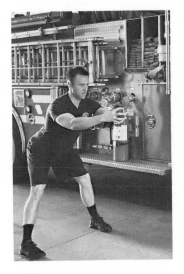

Evan Halquist

I wake up early and immediately jump into a cold plunge for 30 to 60 seconds. It sucks, and then the rest of the day is easier! I do 30 minutes of meditation and breath work, which I look at as mental training. It trains my mind to focus and choose how to respond rather than just react. This is important to me as a husband, father, and firefighter. Then I do some Foundation Training as a warm-up before I strength train. It primes my body and establishes good movement patterns. After my workout, I do 5 minutes of FT as a cooldown to counteract compression and external rotation. I try to do more FT work (just 5 to 10 minutes) throughout the day. It helps give my body and mind energy while keeping me physically and mentally prepared for whatever station or home life has to throw at me. I end my day with a 20-minute meditation in the sauna. This helps to teach my brain and my body to stay relaxed in a stressful environment.

Eating habits-wise, as a firefighter (and human) I think the best thing I can do is not eat too much. I'll limit the time frame I eat each day to only 8 to 12 hours. I fast 24 hours once a week and five days every three months. It boosts the immune system. In terms of what I eat, I try not to complicate it. I eat whole foods, focusing on quality.

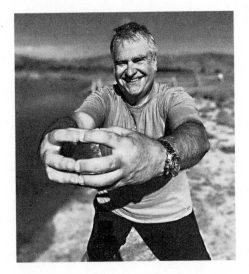

Dr. Pat Helma

When I wake up, the first thing I do is decompression breathing, about 10 breaths, depending on how badly I or the dog has to pee. I practice hip hinging while I brush my teeth, and even do decompression breathing at stoplights, which sometimes freaks people out. I'll practice Foundation Training for about 10 or 15 minutes a day. I take a 25-minute sauna three times a week and employ Buteyko breathing to make sure I stay in the whole time. In terms of exercise, I try to do it outdoors: mountain biking, hiking, skateboarding in the summer. I do some strength training three times a week.

In terms of diet, I try to eat minimally processed, as fresh as I can get, whole foods. I grow a garden in the summer. Unfortunately, I do like beer.

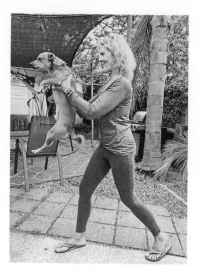

Patti Sheaff

After I wake up and before coffee, I do some deep slow breath work—sometimes 30 Wim Hof breaths before I go surfing. At the beach, I do a Foundation Training warm-up—founder, woodpecker rotations, shoulder trace, and forward fold. To recover from surfing, I'll use my TRX [suspension training system] and more FT. I do a 45-minute infrared sauna almost daily.

I've been using CBD/THC now for a few years, and I feel it helps with recovery and sleep.

I meditate and do qigong on the regular for my physical/spiritual practices, and my diet is pretty clean, not keto but close. Lots of good fats—avocados and salmon. I practice intermittent fasting, but usually just 12 hours.

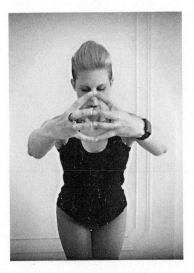

Alli Cost

Diet-wise, I don't eat wheat because I'm legit allergic and will get asthma. Food dyes make me feel terrible, so I try to avoid those at all costs. The most significant health choices I have made in terms of diet are intermittent fasting and whole foods. The intermittent fasting basically because I don't eat anything worthwhile after 7:00 P.M. anyway, and skipping breakfast just makes me feel better somehow. I know some people respond terribly to this diet, so I don't advocate it for everyone, but I was excited to find it. The whole foods approach just means I will eat most anything that was alive or came from the earth recently. Like I pick butter over margarine, grass-fed whole milk over fat-free generic, fancy high percentage dark chocolate over M&M's, local/organic when possible. I think it's important to prepare most of the food you eat for yourself because the love/energy in making it does something to the food. This sounds weird, but it makes sense to me.

I meditate most mornings for 15 to 30 minutes. I prefer guided because I like the idea of learning from someone before sitting in silence with an intention (or mantra). I practice gratitude writing before bed. I used to have a journal and now just write it in an app. My husband/partner has learned to get a kick out of it. As we lie in bed, I list my three things I am thankful for in detail. He answers, "You, you, and you."

For me, breath work is interspersed during the day in 1- to 3-minute bursts. I use the FT decompression breathing or DNS (Dynamic Neuromuscular Stabilization) breathing regularly to "reset" myself several times throughout the day: when waiting for a subway, exercise warm-up or cooldown, and/or when emotionally wound up. These moments feel akin to a mini mediation plus some sit-ups. My brain is clearer, my posture is better, and my core is engaged.

One thing that is relevant to wellness is my people circle. I value my relationships. The people in my life aren't there haphazardly. Being deeply connected to other humans is essential. And this circle defines how we see the world and what we strive to achieve. The ability to be vulnerable, to trust that challenges are opportunities for growth, and relying on deep-rooted loyalty builds the meditation/diet/exercise culture I embrace. All these wellness elements are part of the framework of my relationships. I work out with my friends. My partner and I have similar diets. My career is intertwined with FT because I truly believe in it. Not everyone in my inner circle meditates, but everyone values the benefit and understands that wellness is a priority. If I didn't surround myself with people who are positive and driven to help others, I would not be this way. So I cull those relationships with individuals in my life who show themselves to be selfish or mean.

I practice Foundation Training before every workout for 15 to 30 minutes. Post travel sitting (on plane, car, or train), I will do 5 to 30 minutes, depending on how my body feels. But honestly, I think about it all the time for these micro moments of 5 to 10 seconds, like when I reach into the fridge, clean the cat box, open the front door, and dozens of other little ways throughout the day.

In terms of exercise, I run (3 to 5 miles) a couple times a week. I approach running like I do lifting (form matters, and I am always learning how to integrate other approaches into it). I'll do a high intensity interval workout if running isn't possible. I try to do weight lifting two to three times a week.

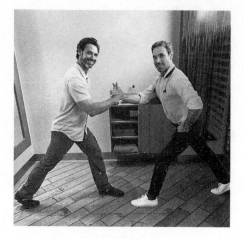

Dr. Ben Carraway

Each day begins with a cold shower and decompression breathing. I won't lie and say that I wake up excited to jump into a cold therapy session because I don't. I confess to having days where I don't want to do it. Switching the temperature from warm to cold is my first act of stoicism for the day, and I do it because it is good for me. I take a cold shower to honor and respect the primitive pathways that keep me alive. I am not a mind within a body, I am a "body," and I salute the autonomic bits. It might sound silly, but if you want your body to serve you, then you should provide it the required stimulus. I know that for my cells to regenerate, they need me to expose them to the cold. Like most normal people, I start my shower warm. I spend the first couple of minutes performing my mental exercises of daily preparation. This is a combination of a private gratitude list and focusing on the day ahead. This ritual is performed under a warm stream of water for the simple reason that I cannot yet do it cold. Setting my psyche to the requirements of the day is key for me. I serve a community as a doctor, and that comes with responsibility. However, before I begin any role outside the house, I am one half of a relationship and also a father. These roles come with duties, and those duties are always changing. To be the best version of myself requires focus and checking the quality of my thoughts so that I am not missing out on life as it is happening.

I perform decompression breathing halfway through my shower. I have a few injuries that include some wear and tear in my lumbar discs, hips, and pubic symphysis, which can be a bit cranky and stiff when I wake up. As little as one minute of decompression breathing expands and relieves any discomfort. I get a fair amount of popping and clicking in my back where the ribs meet my thoracic spine. I love that feeling when breathing becomes more efficient; I can feel small pockets of expansion all over my body, and my shoulders opening and sitting correctly. I like to do my decompression breathing in the morning, because not only am I setting my breathing apparatus up for the day, I am performing my own mini adjustments.

Once my mind and breathing are ready, I switch the temperature to cold . . . It's still uncomfortable. However, one day I aim to be as Zen in the cold as I am comfortable in the warmth. When I first began cold therapy, I'd stay in for 30 seconds. Now I'm up to 2 minutes. While the majority of the benefits I get from exposing my nervous system to the cold are at a cellular level, I do consciously enjoy the heightened sense of alertness, as well as blowing away any sluggish sleepiness to mark a definitive start to the day.

The fundamentals of Foundation Training are woven into the fabric of my day. Through my job as a doctor/teacher, I am reinforcing the FT principle patterns continuously as I go about my business. Every movement that I perform in front of my patients or on the gym floor is an opportunity to teach. If I'm lifting a barbell, a kettlebell, or simply a bag from the floor; I consider it an opportunity to do it well . . .

leading by example. I don't just tell my patients how to discipline their movement, I show them. People come in a variety of forms, and the same is true of our learning styles. However, all humans have mirror neurons, a type of brain cell that helps us learn. During the phenomenally complex processing that our nervous systems perform, the information that our eyes see creates the potential for mimicry. The human brain learns to interpret movement through a process of imitation and is responsible for almost all our complex movements.

The fundamental FT principles have enabled me to be active since 2012, when I discovered Eric's work. As is true of many others, I'm sure, it was injuries that brought me to Foundation Training. Both my own personal impairments and the intellectual curiosity to find the best solutions for my patients. I have what you might describe as skin in the game when it comes to the matter. I was a patient before I became a doctor. Pain is the most powerful tool for discerning what is helpful and what is not. My own practice involves maintaining the integrity of strength patterns around my hips and groin to avoid pain. There is a joint in the front of the human pelvis where two large bones meet, and mine is a bit worn out. That joint is called the pubic symphysis, and mine hurts unless I use Foundation Training to strengthen my hamstrings and adductors. When I say strengthen, I am referring to the mindful practice of feeling the correct structures engage and do the work. If I don't, then the muscles that I overdeveloped through sports attempt to do the job. This is the fundamental process that is so powerful about Foundation Training; you feel stronger when you connect chains of muscles mindfully.

I spent years avoiding rigorous exercise as I studied all the familiar disciplines for an answer. I went from Pilates, physiotherapy, and yoga to chiropractic care, searching for a solution. Throughout the entire course of my degree, I was experimenting with any promising rehabilitation method I could find. Today, thanks to my own practice of Foundation Training, I can dissipate force such that it prevents the stress from overloading my body.

I end every day with a sleep hygiene routine. No screens for one and a half hours before bed, plus four drops of CBD oil, about 40 milligrams, which I take thirty minutes before sleep. I find it helps me recover better and allows me to stay in a deep, restful sleep for longer. Recovery is as essential as any other part of the day.

Eric Goodman

My morning begins early, most often between 5:00 and 6:00 A.M. Water first, at least a liter of it while making a little coffee. On days that I wake up lethargic for any reason, I use an energizing low THC, high CBD strain. I practice decompression breathing, slowly filling the large lobes of my lungs through my nose. I hold the breaths before a slow muscular exhale. I have only a puff or two of cannabis at a time, enough to grease the wheels. I continue decompression breathing practice while I take my dog on a one- to two-hour walk. Other focus points of my walk are the contact points that my feet make with the ground. I focus intently on the entire perimeter of my foot making contact with the ground as I pull my weight away from it. This constant effort to anchor my steps really makes an impact. Often I get lost in the physical sensation of the walk and all of a sudden realize I've been more or less meditating for an hour.

The walk for me is time to connect with nature, rain or shine, no questions. If I have time after the walk to surf, I will. Often, though, I will meet a patient at the beach for a training session in the sand. Work happens in intervals in my life, some days a lot of patients and some days more conference calls and writing. On weeks that I teach certification courses, I feel like I can't eat enough because I talk and talk all day. Days with patients are ridiculously active—moving bodies, training bodies, and manipulating my own body the whole time to be at my best. If I see a lot of patients during the day, I really need to surf or swim in the ocean that evening to decompress differently and allow that energy to process a bit.

Conference calls are often done standing, and if no presentations have to happen, I will take the call for a walk. By 10:00 or 11:00 A.M.,

I have a solid meal of either local fish, beef, or lamb along with vegetables and maybe some sprouted bread or grain. A lot of water all day long. My snacks are dates, potato chips in avocado oil, sprouted cereals with grass-fed whole milk, raw cheese, dark chocolate, or white mulberries pretty much whenever I need a little food.

Bedtime is usually about an hour after a sauna, which is the last thing I do. Look, I know I'm lucky to have a sauna in my house, but it also happens to be the most worthwhile money I've ever paid. Five thousand dollars for a personal Finnish sauna seems pricey. But the mental health, physical relief, and genuine joy it brings will likely save a ton of money on illness and other meds in the future. Find yourself some kind of sauna—it's a worthwhile investment.

Sleep is as good as it gets for a father with a young puppy, a wife in the throes of publishing her own book on human development, and a wonderful toddler daughter. We do our best, I do my best, and the results are damn good so far.

The last thing to remark on is my strong desire to share Foundation Training. If I go a day or two without showing somebody how to help themselves, it seems to really affect me. So as far as addictions are concerned, I know I have them, and the strongest by far is the cherished dopamine hit I get from showing you how good it feels to get better. To get my fix, I teach free community classes and offer assistance to anyone in need. That is how I have built this whole theory into the high-grade human movement that it is.

Gallery

FOUNDATION TRAINING EXERCISES

Following is a gallery of images of the basic Foundation Training exercises. Please note that these photos are for visual reference only. The poses are very subtle. I encourage you to go to www.foundationtraining.com. We have a growing resource of over 1,200 instructors who can teach you in person, or you can use our streaming platform.

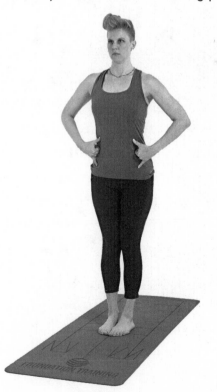

Standing Decompression

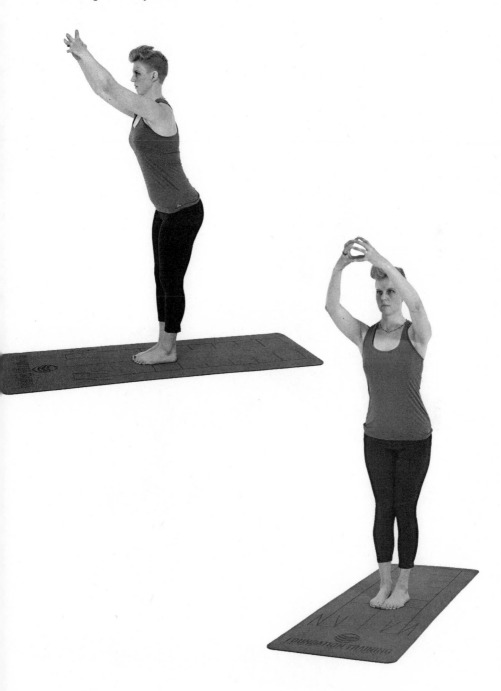

Standing Leg Trace

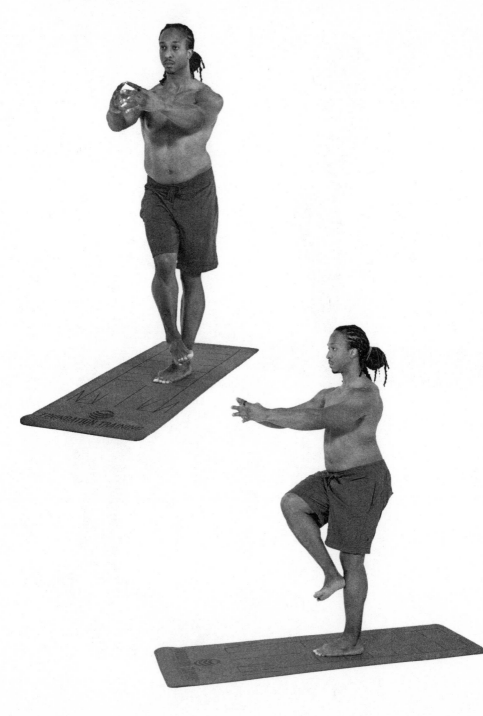

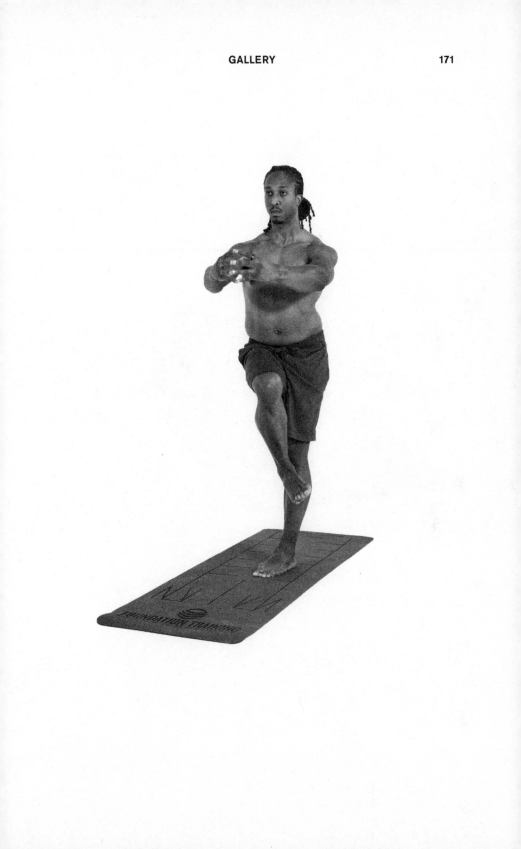

Internal Leg Trace

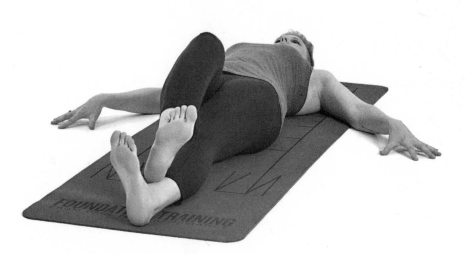

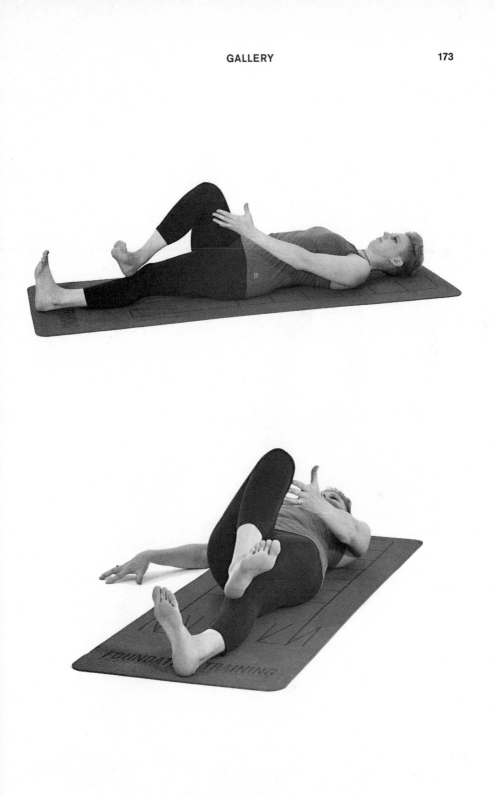

Founder

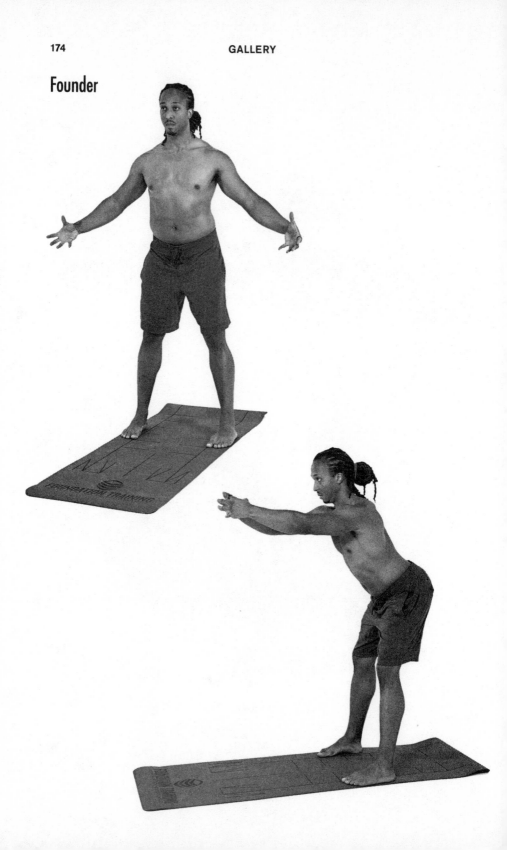

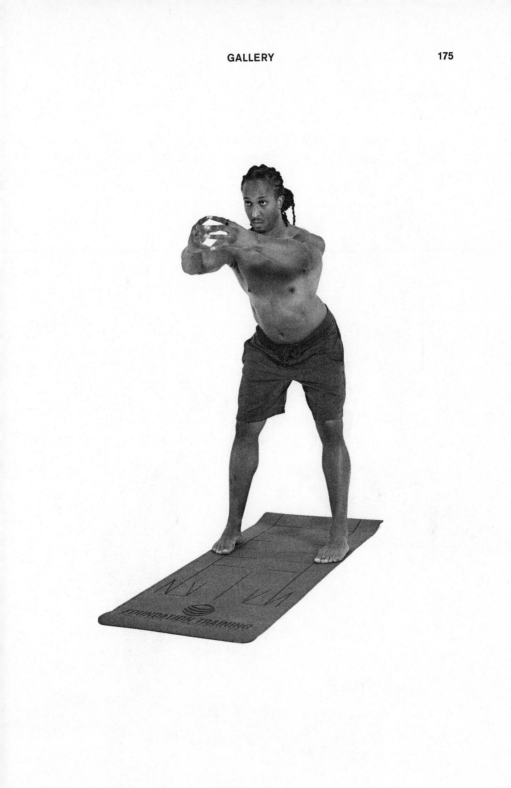

Internal Founder

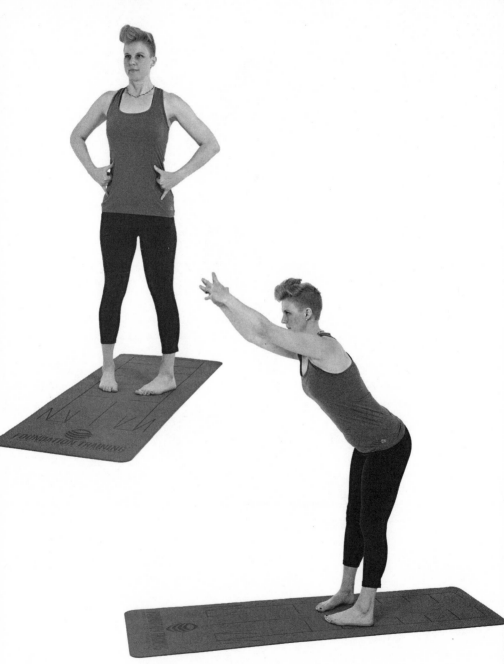

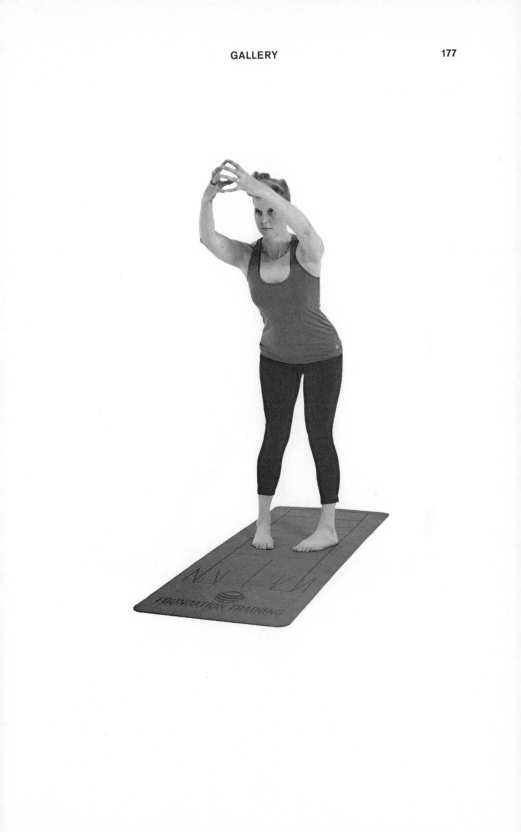

Woodpecker

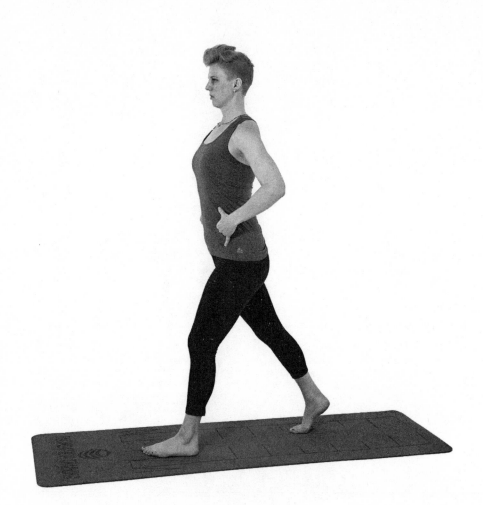

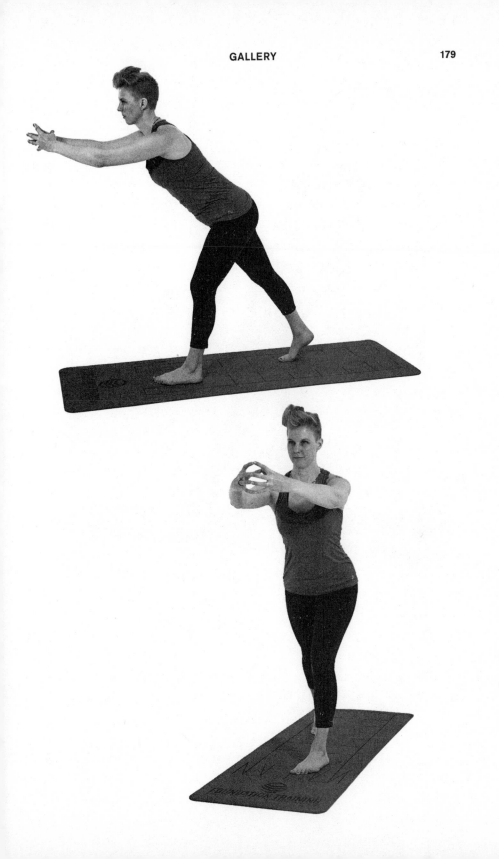

Woodpecker Rotation

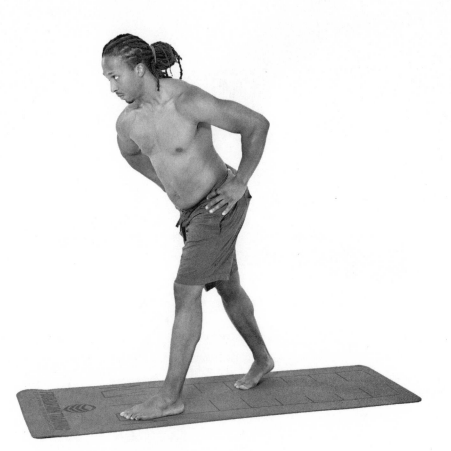

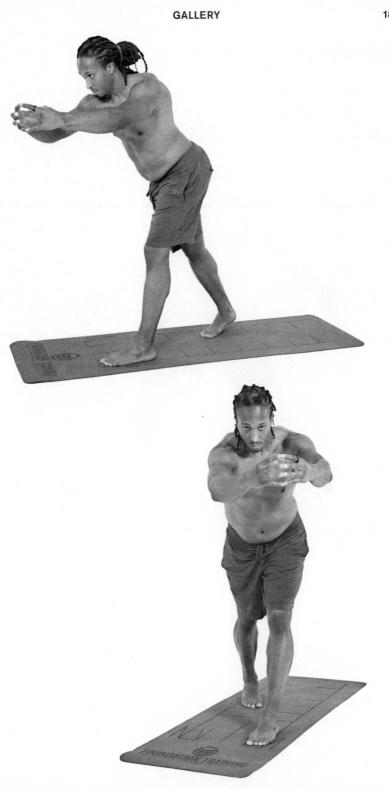

Integrated Hinges

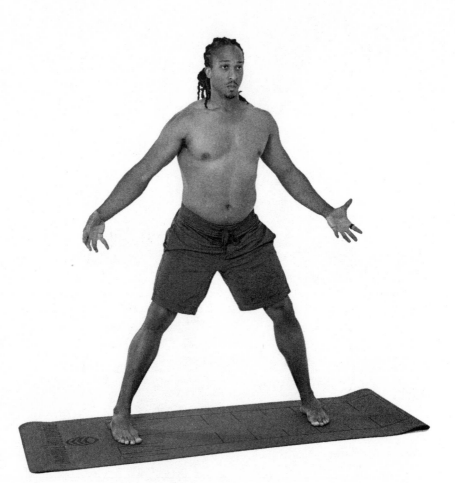

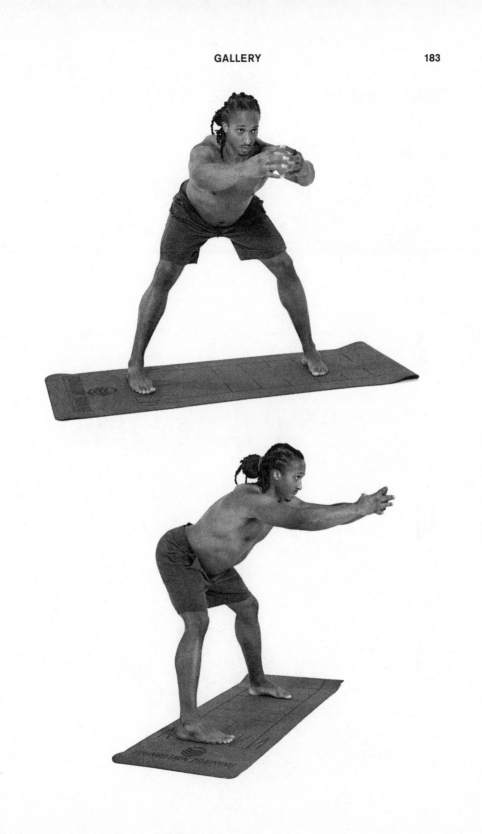

Supine Decompression

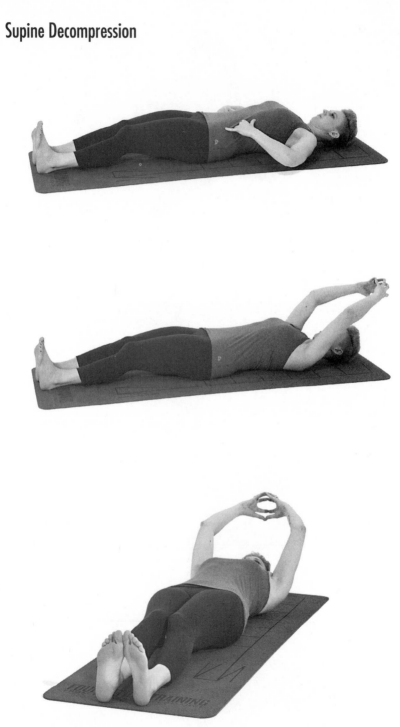

Anchored Bridge

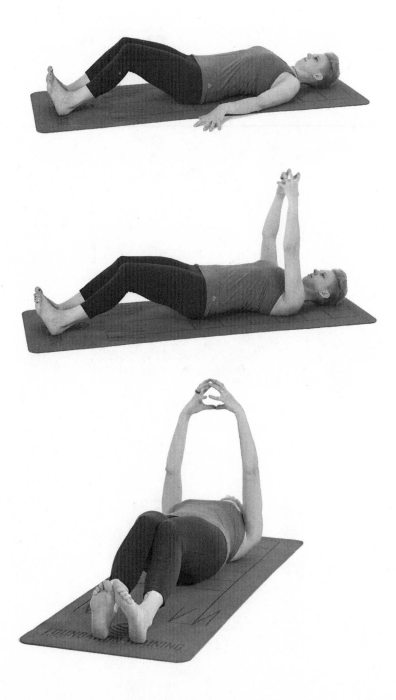

Anchored Back Extension

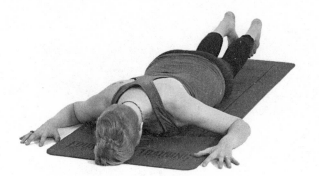

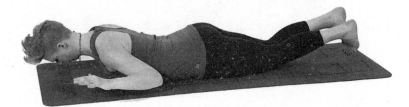

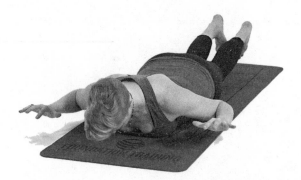

8-Point Plank

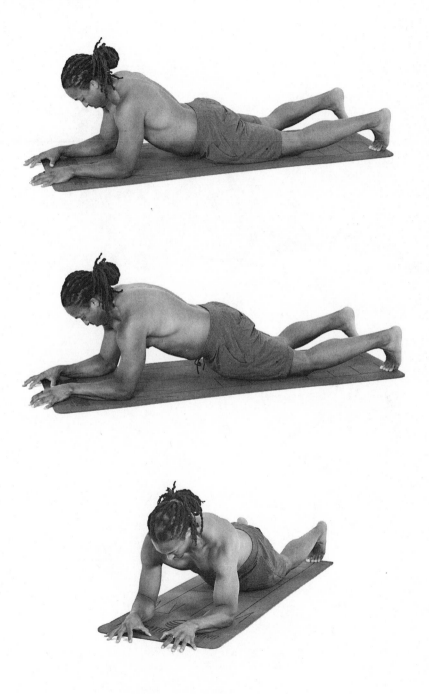

Prone Decompression

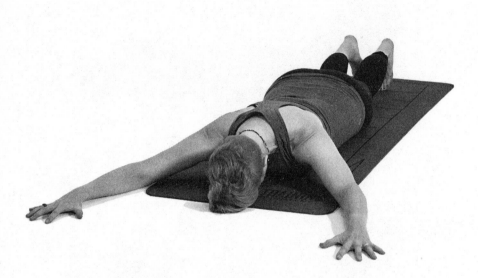

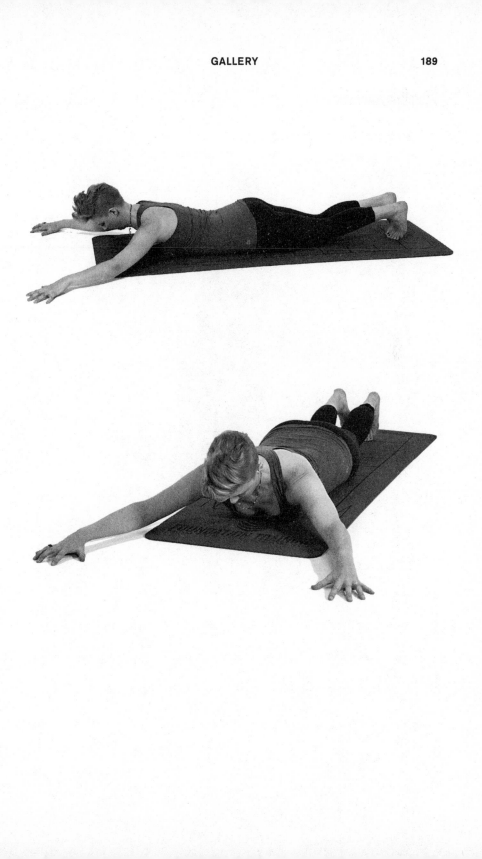

Kneeling Founder

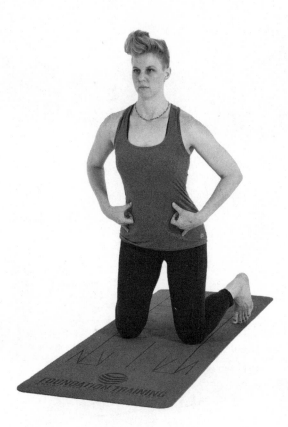

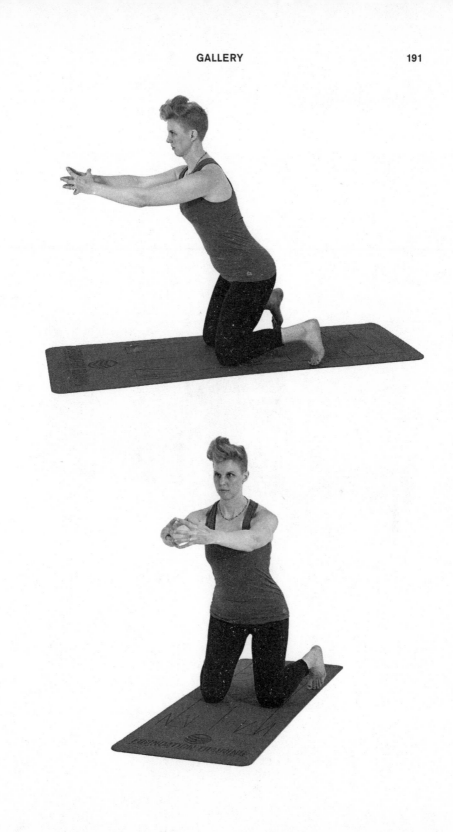

Kneeling Rotation

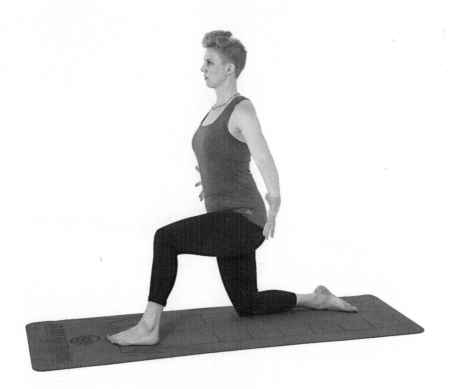

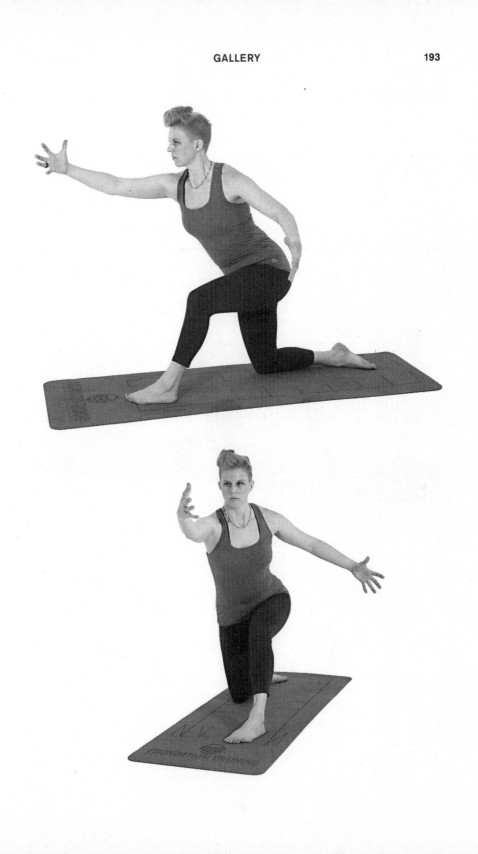

Kneeling Spiral

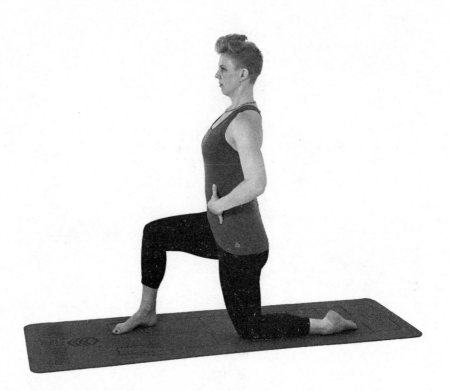

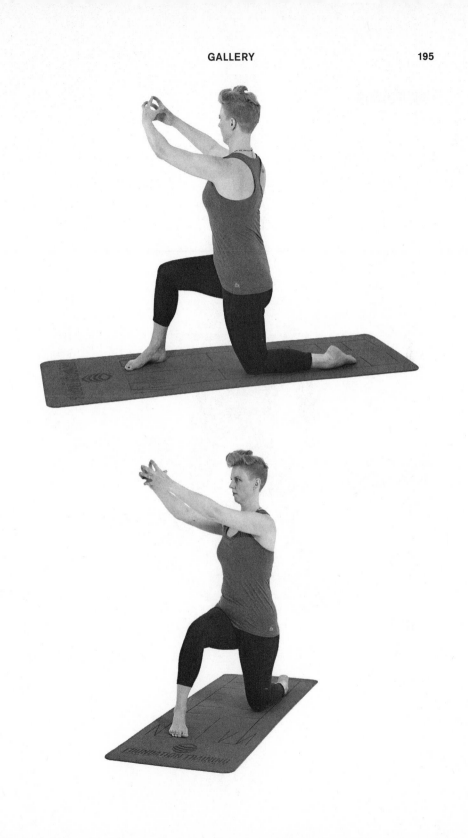

Lateral Hinge

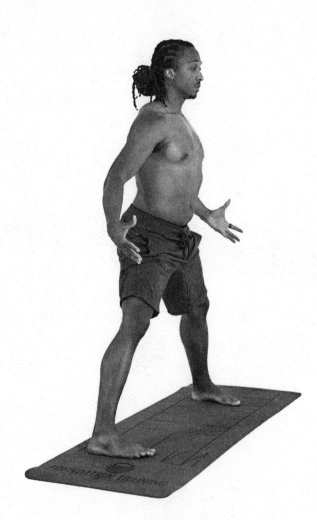

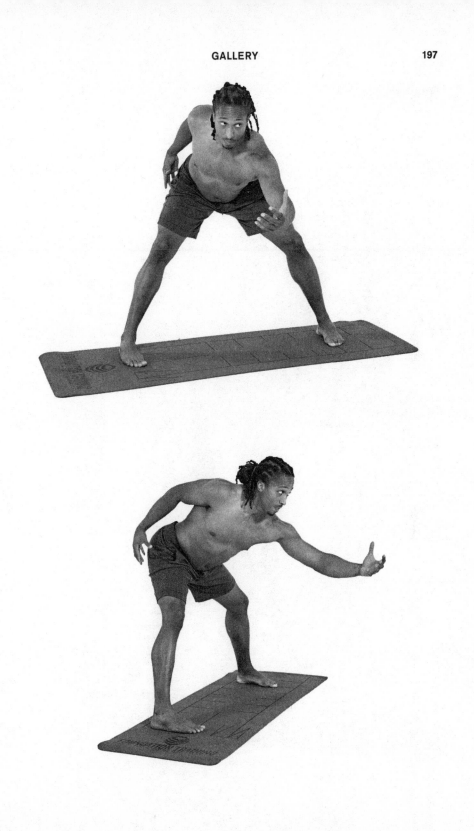

Windmill

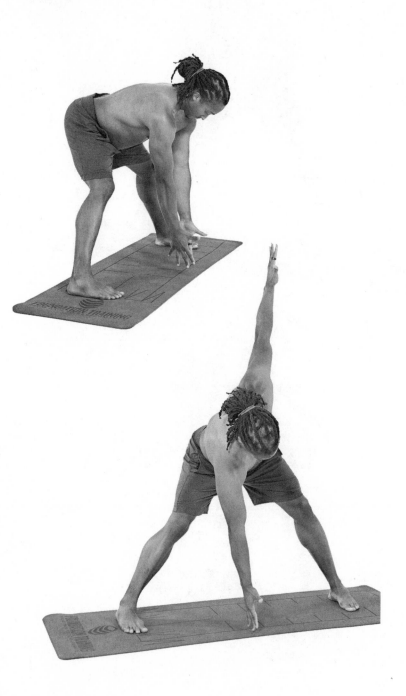

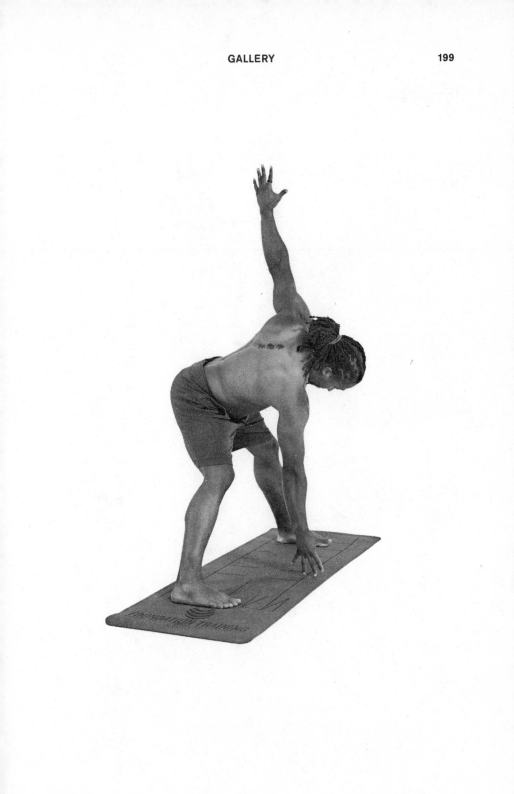

Forward Fold

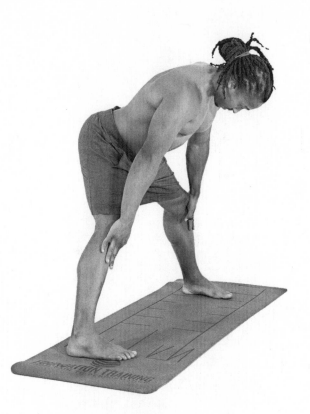

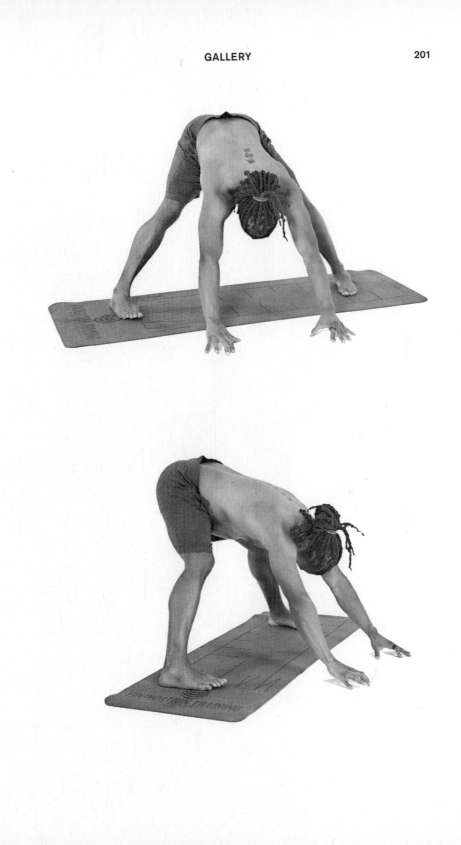

Archer

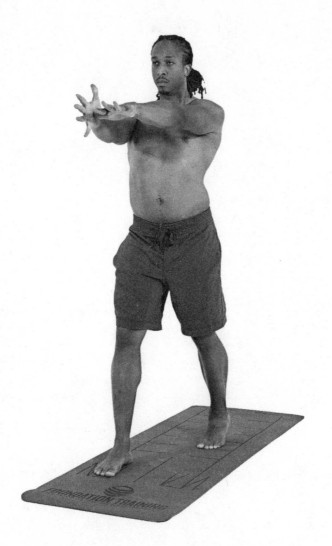

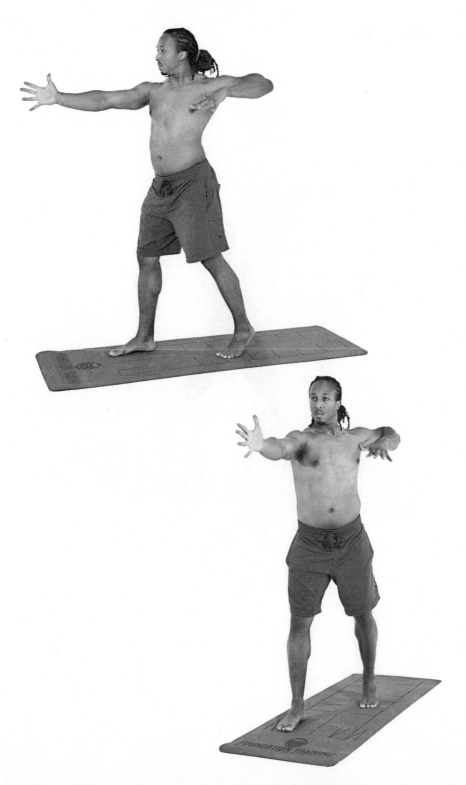

Reverse Archer

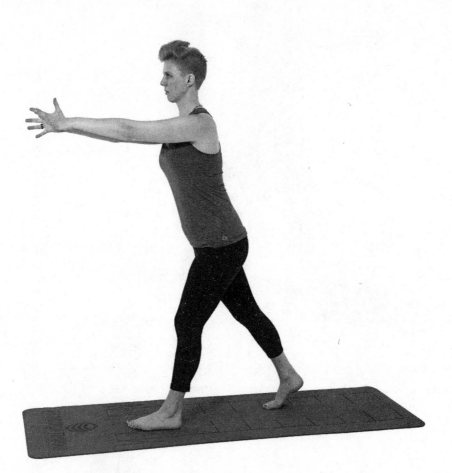

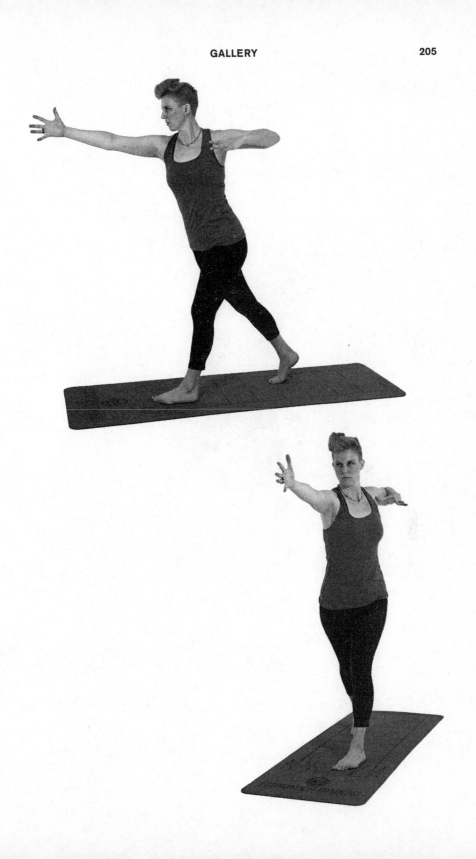

Gorilla Lift

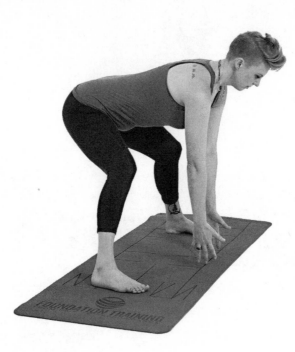

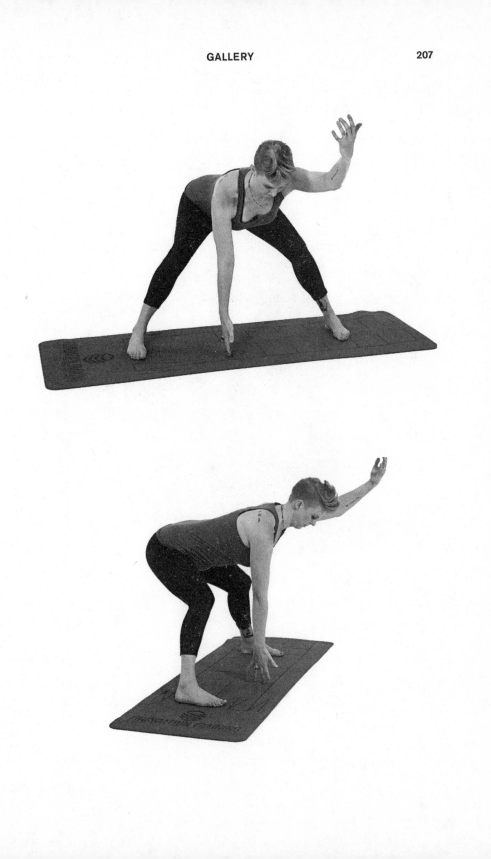

Surf Squat

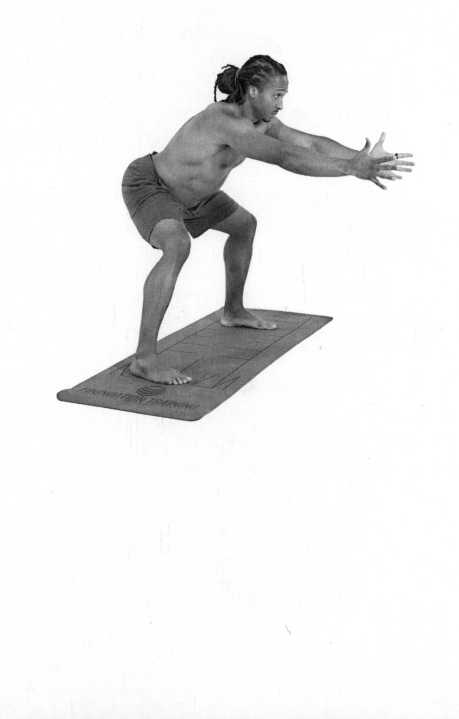

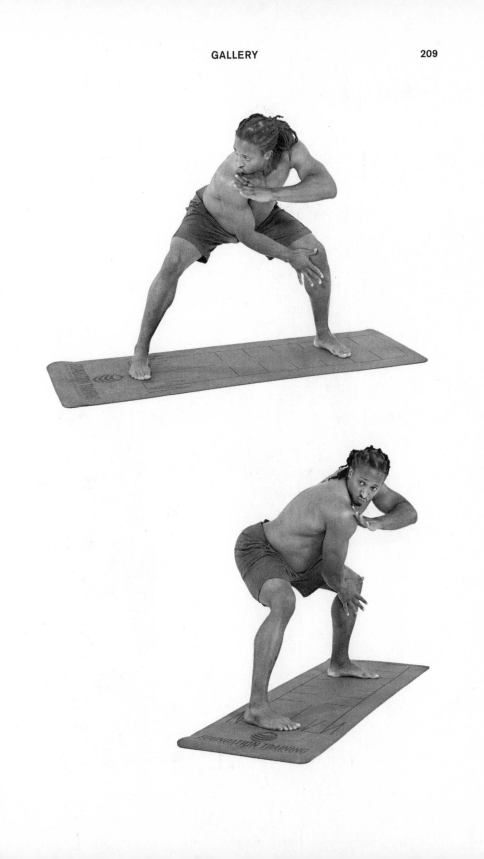

Lunge Decompression

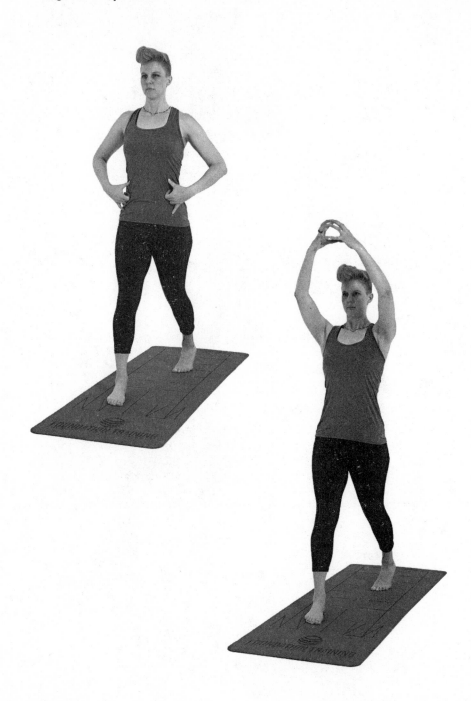

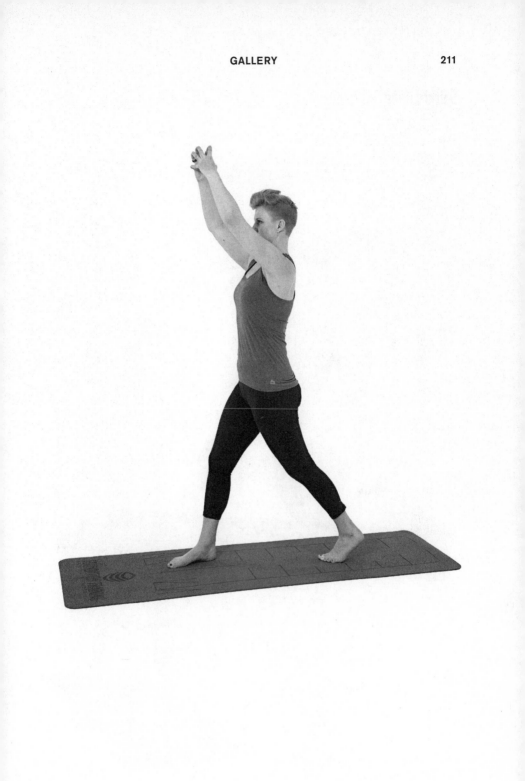

Spiral Lunge

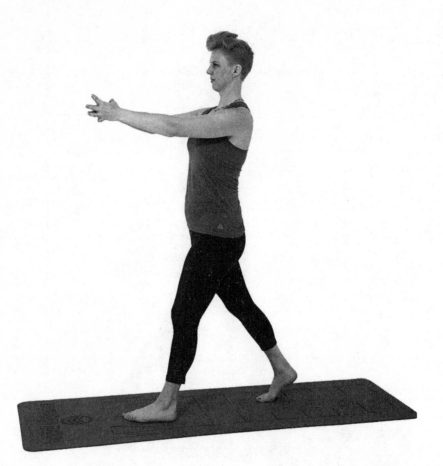

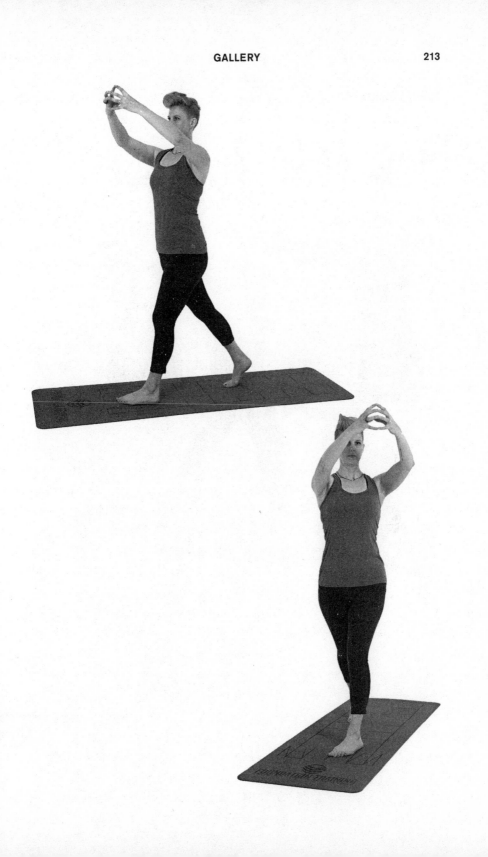

Sphere of Tension

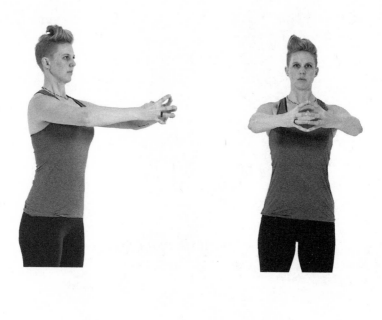

Shoulder Trace

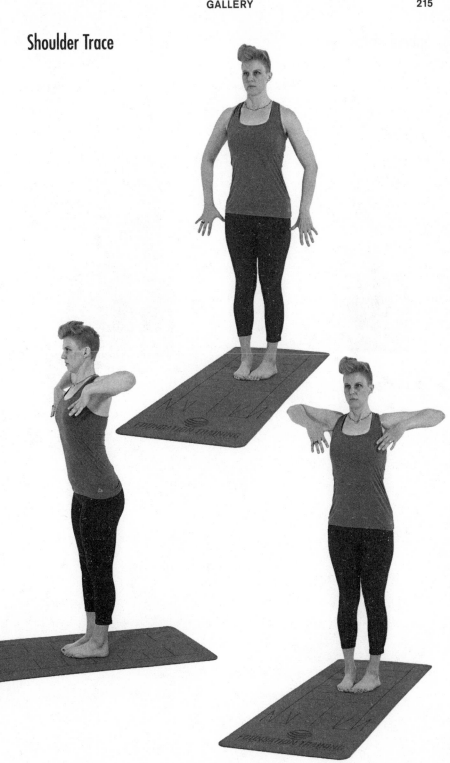

Measuring Sticks

Short Wing

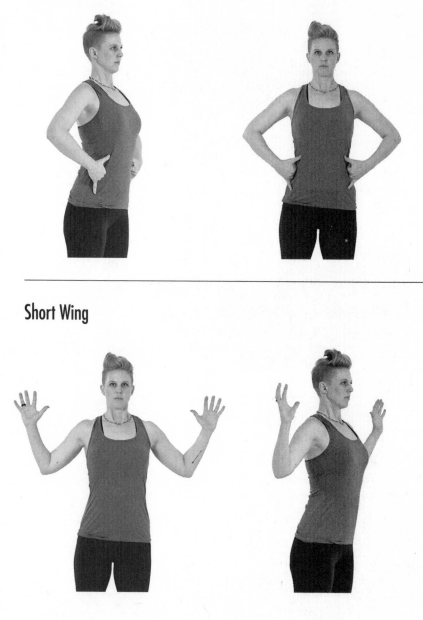

Long Wing

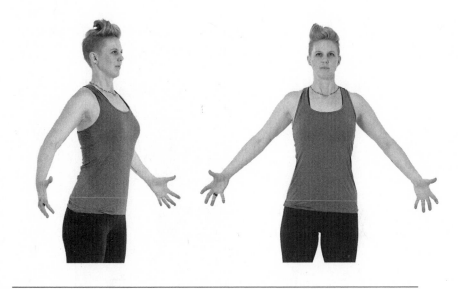

MOFO

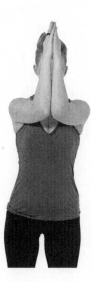
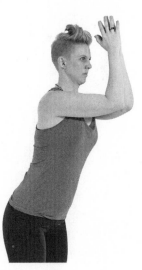

Platter Hands

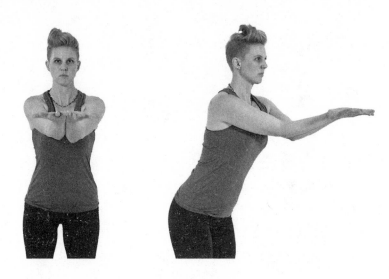

Hip Hugger

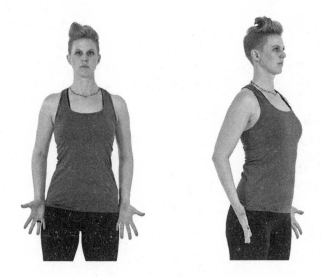

List of Recommended Books and Websites

Blesching, Uwe. *The Cannabis Health Index: Combining the Science of Medical Marijuana with Mindfulness Techniques to Heal 100 Chronic Symptoms and Diseases.* North Atlantic Books, 2015.

Bowman, Katy. *Move Your DNA: Restore Your Health Through Natural Movement,* 2nd ed. Propriometrics Press, 2017.

Millman, Dan. *Way of the Peaceful Warrior: A Book That Changes Lives,* 20th anniversary edition. HJ Kramer, 2006.

Park, Peter, Jesse Lopez Low, and Jussi Lomakka. *Rebound: Regain Strength, Move Effortlessly, Live Without Limits—At Any Age.* Da Capo Lifelong Books, 2018.

Sarno, John. *The Divided Mind: The Epidemic of Mindbody Disorders.* Harper Perennial, 2007.

Sarno, John. *Healing Back Pain: The Mind-Body Connection.* Warner, 1991.

Buteyko Breathing Method: Buteykoclinic.com

Creatine monohydrate for mental and physical strength: www.thorne.com

Independently tested CBD products: https://www.bluesky-cbd.com/

Learn from Joshua Holland: Joshuajholland.com

On the Road to Wellness series with Jessie Salas: https://youtube.com/playlist?list=PLh4zJ2i6o6DLt895znw6B3DYjSOty5uqj

The Progression Project by Erik Antonson: Progressionproject.com

Sample tinctures: PapaandBarkley.com and Kauaihempco.com

Sauna: www.Sauna.com

Sensei Jackson Fortunato: Graciejiujitsuwesthouston.com

Tent Sauna: camping-tent-sauna.com

Tony Blauer's Training Method: Blauerspear.com

Wim Hof Method: wimhofmethod.com

Acknowledgments

Creating this book could not have happened without the help of the following people:

Dr. Dustin DeRyke

Dr. Glenn Goodman

Jessie Salas

Sean Yeager Diamond

Paul Mathieu

Patti Sheaff

Peter Park

Evan Halquist

Dr. Tim Brown

Erik Antonson

Dr. Pat Helma

Jackson Fortunato

Dr. Thomas Hyde

Allison Cost

Dr. Terry Schroeder

Seychelle Webster

Dr. Daniel Kalish

Tony Blauer

Dr. Matt Wiest

Dylan Farr

Dr. Ben Carraway

For your influence and efforts, thank you also to:

Karen Rinaldi

Colin Dickerman

Tal McThenia

Hy Bender

Notes

6   Eighty percent: Vällfors, B. "Acute, Subacute and Chronic Low Back Pain: Clinical Symptoms, Absenteeism and Working Environment." *Scandinavian Journal of Rehabilitation Medicine* supplement no. 11 (Almqvist & Wicksell Periodical Company, 1985): 1–98.

7   Spinal surgeries: Weiss, A. J., and A. Elixhauser. "Trends in Operating Room Procedures in U.S. Hospitals, 2001–2011." HCUP Statistical Brief no. 171 (Rockville, MD: Agency for Healthcare Research and Quality, 2014); Daniell, J. R., and L. O. Orso. "Failed Back Surgery Syndrome: A Review Article." *Asian Spine Journal* 12, no. 2 (2018): 372–79; Weinstein, J. N., et al. "United States' Trends and Regional Variations in Lumbar Spine Surgery: 1992–2003." *Spine* 31, no. 23 (2006): 2707–14.

7   One study: Cited in "Why Back Surgery May Be Unnecessary or Ineffective." Upper Cervical Center of Brandon, October 4, 2018. https://uccenters.com/why-back-surgery-may-be-unnecessary-or-ineffective/.

8   On top: Bernstein, Lenny, and Joel Achenbach, "Drug Overdoses Soared to a Record 93,000 Last Year." *Washington Post*, July 14, 2021. https://www.washingtonpost.com/health/2021/07/14/drug-overdoses-pandemic-2020/.

11 A 2007: Schechter, D., et al. "Outcomes of a Mind-Body Treatment Program for Chronic Back Pain with No Distinct Structural Pathology— A Case Series of Patients Diagnosed and Treated as Tension Myositis Syndrome." *Alternative Therapies in Health and Medicine* 13, no. 5 (2007): 26–35.

71 Study after study: Fitzpatrick, A. "First Responders and PTSD: A Literature Review." *Journal of Emergency Medical Services*, July 28, 2020. https://www.jems.com/administration-and-leadership/first-responders-and

-ptsd-a-literature-review/; "SAMHSA Disaster Technical Assistance Center Supplemental Research Bulletin: First Responders: Behavioral Health Concerns, Emergency Response, and Trauma." Substance Abuse and Mental Health Services Administration, May 2018. https://www.samhsa.gov/sites /default/files/dtac/supplementalresearchbulletin-firstresponders-may2018 .pdf.

71　According to: Abbot, C., et al. "What's Killing Our Medics?" Reviving Responders, April 21, 2015. http://www.revivingresponders.com/original paper.

71　Firefighters face: According to Daniels, R. D., et al. "Mortality and Cancer Incidence in a Pooled Cohort of US Firefighters from San Francisco, Chicago and Philadelphia (1950–2009)." *Occupational and Environmental Medicine* 71, no. 6 (2014): 388–97; Shekhar, A. "Firefighters and Coronary Heart Disease: A Brief History on Research and Analysis." *Fire Engineering*, December 6, 2019. https://www.fireengineering.com /features/firefighters-and-coronary-heart-disease-a-brief-history-on -research-and-analysis/.

72　Those early: Oviir, A. "Here's Why the History of the Sauna Is Deeper than You Might Think." Medium. Estonian Saunas blog, March 18, 2018. https://medium.com/estoniansaunas/heres-why-the-history-of-the -sauna-is-deeper-than-you-might-think-d8e5127a8232.

74　The Kuopio: Kauhanen, J. "Kuopio Ischemic Heart Disease Risk Factor Study." In M. D. Gellman and J. R. Turner, eds., *Encyclopedia of Behavioral Medicine* (New York: Springer, 2013), https://doi.org/10.1007/978–1 –4419–1005–9_328; Laukkanen, J. A., T. Laukkanen, and S. K. Kunutsor. "Cardiovascular and Other Health Benefits of Sauna Bathing: A Review of the Evidence." *Mayo Clinic Proceedings* 93, no. 8 (2018):1111–21.

74　In fact, the study concluded: Laukkanen T., H. Khan, F. Zaccardi, and J. A. Laukkanen. "Association Between Sauna Bathing and Fatal Cardiovascular and All-Cause Mortality Events." *JAMA Internal Medicine* 175, no. 4 (2015): 542–48. doi:10.1001/jamainternmed.2014.8187.

75　our cardiac: Patrick, R. *Sauna Use as an Exercise Mimetic for Heart and Healthspan. Heart Summit 2019.* Found My Fitness, 2019. https://www .foundmyfitness.com/episodes/sauna-heart-presentation.

75　This is: "The Benefit of Regular Sauna Use." Diversified Integrated Sports Clinic, December 19, 2019. https://www.disc-me.com/the-benefit-of -regular-sauna-use/.

82　"stress inoculation training": Ayash, S., et al. "Stress Inoculation in Mice Induces Global Resilience." *Translational Psychiatry* 10 (2020): 200.

82   As an extreme: Kumar, A. "The Grandmaster Diet: How to Lose Weight While Barely Moving." ESPN.com, April 27, 2020. https://www.espn.com /espn/story/_/id/27593253/why-grandmasters-magnus-carlsen-fabiano -caruana-lose-weight-playing-chess.

86   There's also: Lefrançais, E., et al. "The Lung Is a Site of Platelet Biogenesis and a Reservoir for Haematopoietic Progenitors." *Nature* 544 (2017): 105–109. https://www.nature.com/articles/nature21706.

88   When scientists: Learn, J. R. "Science Explains How the Iceman Resists Extreme Cold." Smithsonian.com. Smithsonian Institution, May 22, 2018. https://www.smithsonianmag.com/science-nature/science-explains-how -iceman-resists-extreme-cold-180969134/.

95   We don't: Lawler, A. "Oldest Evidence of Marijuana Use Discovered in 2500-Year-Old Cemetery in Peaks of Western China." *Science*, June 12, 2019. https://www.sciencemag.org/news/2019/06/oldest-evidence-marijuana -use-discovered-2500-year-old-cemetery-peaks-western-china.

103 When we: Bagar, T. "The Endocannabinoid System and Stress Response Implication in Fatigue and Burn-out." Fundación CANNA: Scientific studies and cannabis testing.

103 What's more: Hill, M.N., and S. Patel. "Endocannabinoid Signaling and Stress Resilience." In A. Chen, ed., *Stress Resilience* (New York: Academic Press, 2019), 349–62.

106 In some cases: Russo, E. B. "Clinical Endocannabinoid Deficiency Reconsidered: Current Research Supports the Theory in Migraine, Fibromyalgia, Irritable Bowel, and Other Treatment-Resistant Syndromes." *Cannabis and Cannabinoid Research* 1, no. 1 (2016): 154–65.

105 According to: Earlenbaugh, E. "Clinical Endocannabinoid Deficiency: When Does It Happen and Why?" *The Cannigma*, May 16, 2021. https:// cannigma.com/physiology/clinical-endocannabinoid-deficiency-when -does-it-happen-and-why/.

108 Recent science: Charytoniuk, T., et al. "Can Physical Activity Support the Endocannabinoid System in the Preventive and Therapeutic Approach to Neurological Disorders?" *International Journal of Molecular Sciences* 21, no.12 (2020): 4221.

108 In one: Crombie, K. M., et al. "Endocannabinoid and Opioid System Interactions in Exercise-Induced Hypoalgesia." *Pain Medicine* 19, no. 1 (2018): 118–23.

118 [W]ith millions: Knox, R. "The Endocannabinoid System and the Revolution of One," TEDxPortland. YouTube, 2019. https://www.youtube.com /watch?v=oJbOQ9P2NYQ.

119 Then came: Green, M. "Reefer Madness! The Twisted History of America's Marijuana Laws." KQED, January 5, 2018. https://www.kqed.org/low down/24153/reefer-madness-the-twisted-history-of-americas-weed-laws.

119 In doing: Fishbein, M. "Federal Regulation of Medicinal Use of Cannabis." *JAMA* 108 (1937):1543–44; Okie, S. "Medical Marijuana and the Supreme Court." *New England Journal of Medicine* 353 (2005): 648–51.

122 If you're: "Pot Smokers Can Maybe Breathe a Little Easier." Harvard Health Publishing, *Staying Healthy*, March 1, 2012. https://www.health .harvard.edu/staying-healthy/pot-smokers-can-maybe-breathe-a-little -easier; Ribeiro, L., and P. W. Ind. "Marijuana and the Lung: Hysteria or Cause for Concern?" *Breathe* 14, no. 3 (2018): 196–205.

125 In a: Woolridge, E., S. Barton, J. Samuel, J. Osorio, A. Dougherty, and A. Holdcroft. "Cannabis Use in HIV for Pain and Other Medical Symptoms," *Journal of Pain and Symptom Management* 29, no. 4, 2005: 358–67, ISSN 0885–3924, https://doi.org/10.1016/j.jpainsymman.2004.07.011 (https:// www.sciencedirect.com/science/article/pii/S0885392405000631).

125 As an: Russo, E. B. "Cannabinoids in the Management of Difficult to Treat Pain." *Therapeutics and Clinical Risk Management* 4, no. 1 (2008): 245–59.

125 THC is: Currais, A., et al. "Amyloid Proteotoxicity Initiates an Inflammatory Response Blocked by Cannabinoids." *Aging and Mechanisms of Disease* 2, no. 1: 16012 (2016).

129 Or comedian: MPI Media Group. "George Carlin: 40 Years of Comedy Online: Vimeo On Demand." Vimeo, 1997. https://vimeo.com/ondemand /40yearsofcomedy.

129 In terms: Pandika, M. "Does Weed Enhance Creativity? A Doctor Weighs In." Mic, October 21, 2020. https://www.mic.com/p/does-weed-enhance -creativity-a-doctor-weighs-in-39792615.

130 The study: Schafer, G., et al. "Investigating the Interaction Between Schizotypy, Divergent Thinking and Cannabis Use." *Consciousness and Cognition* 21, no. 1 (2012): 292–98.

130 Another 2010: Morgan, C. J. A., E. Rothwell, H. Atkinson, O. Mason, and H. V. Curran. "Hyper-Priming in Cannabis Users: A Naturalistic Study of the Effects of Cannabis on Semantic Memory Function," *Psychiatry Research* 176, nos. 2–3, 2010: 213–18, ISSN 0165–1781, https://doi .org/10.1016/j.psychres.2008.09.002.

132 In fact: Alshaarawy, O., and J. C. Anthony. "Are Cannabis Users Less Likely to Gain Weight? Results from a National 3-Year Prospective Study." *International Journal of Epidemiology* 48, no. 5 (2019): 1695–1700.

133 In one: Nguyen, T. "Working Out with Weed." *Nature News*, August 28, 2019. https://www.nature.com/articles/d41586–019–02529–0.

Art Credits

Exercise Photos (Gallery): Paul Mathieu
Illustrations (Chapter 2): Dr. Dustin DeRyke

INDIVIDUAL PHOTOS:

Seychelle Webster: Benjamin Thacker
Alli Cost: Jovis DePognon
Tony Blauer: Jesse Blauer
Jackson Fortunato: photo courtesy of Jackson Fortunato
Evan Halquist: Jessie Salas
Jessie Salas: Giancarlo Beroldo
Ben Carraway: Jessie Salas
Erik Antonson: Sarah Antonson
Patti Sheaff: Price Marshall

Index

Page numbers in italics indicate images

About the Author

DR. ERIC GOODMAN has spent his professional life learning from his patients and from his own symptoms. Educated originally as a Doctor of Chiropractic, Eric began quickly paving his own path in pain management through specific movements called Foundation Training.

Dr. Goodman has brought innovation, compassion, and action to the chronic pain community, and continues to work tirelessly to improve the lives of those willing to put in the effort to help themselves heal.

In addition to *Foundations of Health*, Eric has written *Foundation* (2011) and *True to Form* (2016), and coauthored *Shaping Your Baby's Foundation* with his wife, Jen Goodman, in 2021.

You can learn more about his work at FoundationTraining.com.